Food and Exercise Journal 2016
Weekly Food & Workout Diary

Fierce & Fabulous

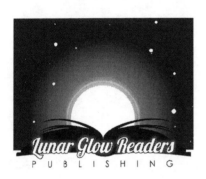

January 2016

Friday 1

Breakfast | Lunch | Dinner

WorkOut Time
● LOWER BODY | ● CORE | ● UPPER BODY | ● CARDIO | ● STRETCH | ● OTHER

GLASSES OF WATER
STRESS 1 2 3 4 5 6 7 8 9 10

Saturday 2

Breakfast | Lunch | Dinner

WorkOut Time
● LOWER BODY | ● CORE | ● UPPER BODY | ● CARDIO | ● STRETCH | ● OTHER

GLASSES OF WATER
STRESS 1 2 3 4 5 6 7 8 9 10

Sunday 3

Breakfast | Lunch | Dinner

WorkOut Time
● LOWER BODY | ● CORE | ● UPPER BODY | ● CARDIO | ● STRETCH | ● OTHER

GLASSES OF WATER
STRESS 1 2 3 4 5 6 7 8 9 10

Notes

Monday 4

Breakfast   Lunch   Dinner

WorkOut   ● LOWER BODY   ● CORE   ● UPPER BODY   ● CARDIO   ● STRETCH   ● OTHER
Time

GLASSES OF WATER
STRESS   1 2 3 4 5 6 7 8 9 10

Tuesday 5

Breakfast   Lunch   Dinner

WorkOut   ● LOWER BODY   ● CORE   ● UPPER BODY   ● CARDIO   ● STRETCH   ● OTHER
Time

GLASSES OF WATER
STRESS   1 2 3 4 5 6 7 8 9 10

Wednesday 6

Breakfast   Lunch   Dinner

WorkOut   ● LOWER BODY   ● CORE   ● UPPER BODY   ● CARDIO   ● STRETCH   ● OTHER
Time

GLASSES OF WATER
STRESS   1 2 3 4 5 6 7 8 9 10

Thursday 7

Breakfast   Lunch   Dinner

WorkOut   ● LOWER BODY   ● CORE   ● UPPER BODY   ● CARDIO   ● STRETCH   ● OTHER
Time

GLASSES OF WATER
STRESS   1 2 3 4 5 6 7 8 9 10

Friday 8

Breakfast　　　Lunch　　　Dinner

WorkOut Time
● LOWER BODY　● CORE　● UPPER BODY　● CARDIO　● STRETCH　● OTHER

GLASSES OF WATER

STRESS 1 2 3 4 5 6 7 8 9 10

Saturday 9

Breakfast　　　Lunch　　　Dinner

WorkOut Time
● LOWER BODY　● CORE　● UPPER BODY　● CARDIO　● STRETCH　● OTHER

GLASSES OF WATER

STRESS 1 2 3 4 5 6 7 8 9 10

Sunday 10

Breakfast　　　Lunch　　　Dinner

WorkOut Time
● LOWER BODY　● CORE　● UPPER BODY　● CARDIO　● STRETCH　● OTHER

GLASSES OF WATER

STRESS 1 2 3 4 5 6 7 8 9 10

Notes

January 2016

Monday 11

Breakfast | Lunch | Dinner
_____
_____
_____
_____

WorkOut ● LOWER BODY ● CORE ● UPPER BODY ● CARDIO ● STRETCH ● OTHER
Time [ ] [ ] [ ] [ ] [ ] [ ]

GLASSES OF WATER
STRESS 1 2 3 4 5 6 7 8 9 10

Tuesday 12

Breakfast | Lunch | Dinner
_____
_____
_____
_____

WorkOut ● LOWER BODY ● CORE ● UPPER BODY ● CARDIO ● STRETCH ● OTHER
Time [ ] [ ] [ ] [ ] [ ] [ ]

GLASSES OF WATER
STRESS 1 2 3 4 5 6 7 8 9 10

Wednesday 13

Breakfast | Lunch | Dinner
_____
_____
_____
_____

WorkOut ● LOWER BODY ● CORE ● UPPER BODY ● CARDIO ● STRETCH ● OTHER
Time [ ] [ ] [ ] [ ] [ ] [ ]

GLASSES OF WATER
STRESS 1 2 3 4 5 6 7 8 9 10

Thursday 14

Breakfast | Lunch | Dinner
_____
_____
_____
_____

WorkOut ● LOWER BODY ● CORE ● UPPER BODY ● CARDIO ● STRETCH ● OTHER
Time [ ] [ ] [ ] [ ] [ ] [ ]

GLASSES OF WATER
STRESS 1 2 3 4 5 6 7 8 9 10

January 2016

Friday 15

Breakfast **Lunch** **Dinner**

WorkOut Time
● LOWER BODY ● CORE ● UPPER BODY ● CARDIO ● STRETCH ● OTHER

GLASSES OF WATER
STRESS 1 2 3 4 5 6 7 8 9 10

Saturday 16

Breakfast **Lunch** **Dinner**

WorkOut Time
● LOWER BODY ● CORE ● UPPER BODY ● CARDIO ● STRETCH ● OTHER

GLASSES OF WATER
STRESS 1 2 3 4 5 6 7 8 9 10

Sunday 17

Breakfast **Lunch** **Dinner**

WorkOut Time
● LOWER BODY ● CORE ● UPPER BODY ● CARDIO ● STRETCH ● OTHER

GLASSES OF WATER
STRESS 1 2 3 4 5 6 7 8 9 10

Notes

January 2016

Monday 18

Breakfast | Lunch | Dinner

WorkOut ● LOWER BODY ● CORE ● UPPER BODY ● CARDIO ● STRETCH ● OTHER
Time [ ] [ ] [ ] [ ] [ ] [ ]

GLASSES OF WATER
STRESS 1 2 3 4 5 6 7 8 9 10

Tuesday 19

Breakfast | Lunch | Dinner

WorkOut ● LOWER BODY ● CORE ● UPPER BODY ● CARDIO ● STRETCH ● OTHER
Time [ ] [ ] [ ] [ ] [ ] [ ]

GLASSES OF WATER
STRESS 1 2 3 4 5 6 7 8 9 10

Wednesday 20

Breakfast | Lunch | Dinner

WorkOut ● LOWER BODY ● CORE ● UPPER BODY ● CARDIO ● STRETCH ● OTHER
Time [ ] [ ] [ ] [ ] [ ] [ ]

GLASSES OF WATER
STRESS 1 2 3 4 5 6 7 8 9 10

Thursday 21

Breakfast | Lunch | Dinner

WorkOut ● LOWER BODY ● CORE ● UPPER BODY ● CARDIO ● STRETCH ● OTHER
Time [ ] [ ] [ ] [ ] [ ] [ ]

GLASSES OF WATER
STRESS 1 2 3 4 5 6 7 8 9 10

Friday
22

Breakfast   Lunch   Dinner

WorkOut ● LOWER BODY ● CORE ● UPPER BODY ● CARDIO ● STRETCH ● OTHER
Time

GLASSES OF WATER
STRESS 1 2 3 4 5 6 7 8 9 10

Saturday
23

Breakfast   Lunch   Dinner

WorkOut ● LOWER BODY ● CORE ● UPPER BODY ● CARDIO ● STRETCH ● OTHER
Time

GLASSES OF WATER
STRESS 1 2 3 4 5 6 7 8 9 10

Sunday
24

Breakfast   Lunch   Dinner

WorkOut ● LOWER BODY ● CORE ● UPPER BODY ● CARDIO ● STRETCH ● OTHER
Time

GLASSES OF WATER
STRESS 1 2 3 4 5 6 7 8 9 10

Notes

Monday 25

Breakfast	Lunch	Dinner

WorkOut Time ● LOWER BODY ● CORE ● UPPER BODY ● CARDIO ● STRETCH ● OTHER

GLASSES OF WATER
STRESS 1 2 3 4 5 6 7 8 9 10

Tuesday 26

Breakfast	Lunch	Dinner

WorkOut Time ● LOWER BODY ● CORE ● UPPER BODY ● CARDIO ● STRETCH ● OTHER

GLASSES OF WATER
STRESS 1 2 3 4 5 6 7 8 9 10

Wednesday 27

Breakfast	Lunch	Dinner

WorkOut Time ● LOWER BODY ● CORE ● UPPER BODY ● CARDIO ● STRETCH ● OTHER

GLASSES OF WATER
STRESS 1 2 3 4 5 6 7 8 9 10

Thursday 28

Breakfast	Lunch	Dinner

WorkOut Time ● LOWER BODY ● CORE ● UPPER BODY ● CARDIO ● STRETCH ● OTHER

GLASSES OF WATER
STRESS 1 2 3 4 5 6 7 8 9 10

Friday 29

Breakfast	Lunch	Dinner

WorkOut ● LOWER BODY ● CORE ● UPPER BODY ● CARDIO ● STRETCH ● OTHER
Time

GLASSES OF WATER

STRESS 1 2 3 4 5 6 7 8 9 10

Saturday 30

Breakfast	Lunch	Dinner

WorkOut ● LOWER BODY ● CORE ● UPPER BODY ● CARDIO ● STRETCH ● OTHER
Time

GLASSES OF WATER

STRESS 1 2 3 4 5 6 7 8 9 10

Sunday 31

Breakfast	Lunch	Dinner

WorkOut ● LOWER BODY ● CORE ● UPPER BODY ● CARDIO ● STRETCH ● OTHER
Time

GLASSES OF WATER

STRESS 1 2 3 4 5 6 7 8 9 10

This Month's Measurements:

Waist
Neck
Biceps
Chest
Hips
Thighs

Month Progress Report

Current Weight:

Notes:

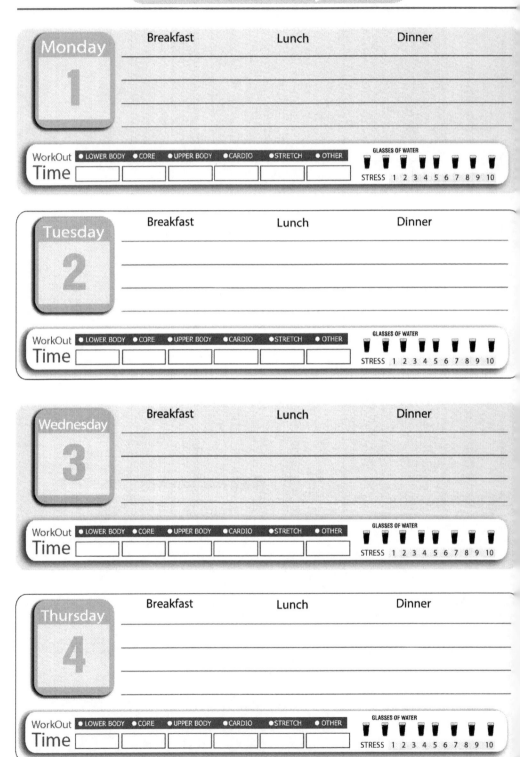

February 2016

Monday 1

Breakfast Lunch Dinner

WorkOut ● LOWER BODY ● CORE ● UPPER BODY ● CARDIO ● STRETCH ● OTHER
Time

GLASSES OF WATER
STRESS 1 2 3 4 5 6 7 8 9 10

Tuesday 2

Breakfast Lunch Dinner

WorkOut ● LOWER BODY ● CORE ● UPPER BODY ● CARDIO ● STRETCH ● OTHER
Time

GLASSES OF WATER
STRESS 1 2 3 4 5 6 7 8 9 10

Wednesday 3

Breakfast Lunch Dinner

WorkOut ● LOWER BODY ● CORE ● UPPER BODY ● CARDIO ● STRETCH ● OTHER
Time

GLASSES OF WATER
STRESS 1 2 3 4 5 6 7 8 9 10

Thursday 4

Breakfast Lunch Dinner

WorkOut ● LOWER BODY ● CORE ● UPPER BODY ● CARDIO ● STRETCH ● OTHER
Time

GLASSES OF WATER
STRESS 1 2 3 4 5 6 7 8 9 10

Friday
5

Breakfast Lunch Dinner

WorkOut
Time

● LOWER BODY ● CORE ● UPPER BODY ● CARDIO ● STRETCH ● OTHER

GLASSES OF WATER

STRESS 1 2 3 4 5 6 7 8 9 10

Saturday
6

Breakfast Lunch Dinner

WorkOut
Time

● LOWER BODY ● CORE ● UPPER BODY ● CARDIO ● STRETCH ● OTHER

GLASSES OF WATER

STRESS 1 2 3 4 5 6 7 8 9 10

Sunday
7

Breakfast Lunch Dinner

WorkOut
Time

● LOWER BODY ● CORE ● UPPER BODY ● CARDIO ● STRETCH ● OTHER

GLASSES OF WATER

STRESS 1 2 3 4 5 6 7 8 9 10

Notes

February 2016

Monday 8

Breakfast — Lunch — Dinner

WorkOut Time — ● LOWER BODY ● CORE ● UPPER BODY ● CARDIO ● STRETCH ● OTHER

GLASSES OF WATER

STRESS 1 2 3 4 5 6 7 8 9 10

Tuesday 9

Breakfast — Lunch — Dinner

WorkOut Time — ● LOWER BODY ● CORE ● UPPER BODY ● CARDIO ● STRETCH ● OTHER

GLASSES OF WATER

STRESS 1 2 3 4 5 6 7 8 9 10

Wednesday 10

Breakfast — Lunch — Dinner

WorkOut Time — ● LOWER BODY ● CORE ● UPPER BODY ● CARDIO ● STRETCH ● OTHER

GLASSES OF WATER

STRESS 1 2 3 4 5 6 7 8 9 10

Thursday 11

Breakfast — Lunch — Dinner

WorkOut Time — ● LOWER BODY ● CORE ● UPPER BODY ● CARDIO ● STRETCH ● OTHER

GLASSES OF WATER

STRESS 1 2 3 4 5 6 7 8 9 10

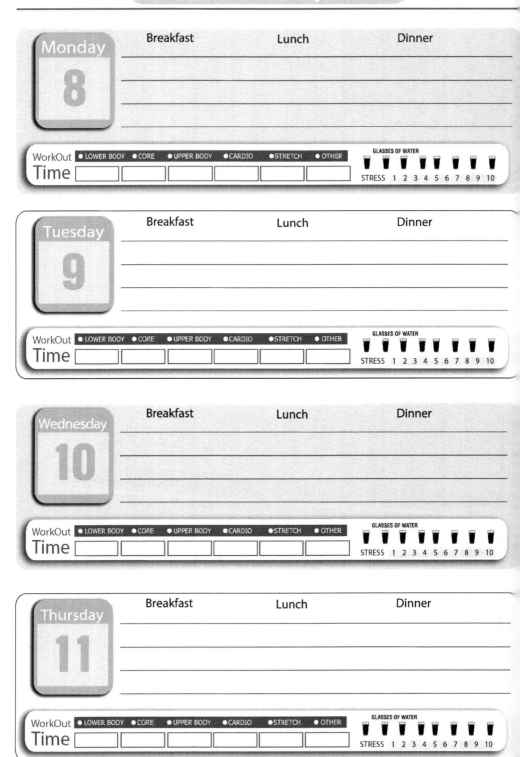

Friday 12

Breakfast	Lunch	Dinner

WorkOut ● LOWER BODY ● CORE ● UPPER BODY ● CARDIO ● STRETCH ● OTHER
Time

GLASSES OF WATER
STRESS 1 2 3 4 5 6 7 8 9 10

Saturday 13

Breakfast	Lunch	Dinner

WorkOut ● LOWER BODY ● CORE ● UPPER BODY ● CARDIO ● STRETCH ● OTHER
Time

GLASSES OF WATER
STRESS 1 2 3 4 5 6 7 8 9 10

Sunday 14

Breakfast	Lunch	Dinner

WorkOut ● LOWER BODY ● CORE ● UPPER BODY ● CARDIO ● STRETCH ● OTHER
Time

GLASSES OF WATER
STRESS 1 2 3 4 5 6 7 8 9 10

Notes

February 2016

Monday 15

Breakfast	Lunch	Dinner

WorkOut ● LOWER BODY ● CORE ● UPPER BODY ● CARDIO ● STRETCH ● OTHER

Time ☐ ☐ ☐ ☐ ☐ ☐

GLASSES OF WATER

STRESS 1 2 3 4 5 6 7 8 9 10

Tuesday 16

Breakfast	Lunch	Dinner

WorkOut ● LOWER BODY ● CORE ● UPPER BODY ● CARDIO ● STRETCH ● OTHER

Time ☐ ☐ ☐ ☐ ☐ ☐

GLASSES OF WATER

STRESS 1 2 3 4 5 6 7 8 9 10

Wednesday 17

Breakfast	Lunch	Dinner

WorkOut ● LOWER BODY ● CORE ● UPPER BODY ● CARDIO ● STRETCH ● OTHER

Time ☐ ☐ ☐ ☐ ☐ ☐

GLASSES OF WATER

STRESS 1 2 3 4 5 6 7 8 9 10

Thursday 18

Breakfast	Lunch	Dinner

WorkOut ● LOWER BODY ● CORE ● UPPER BODY ● CARDIO ● STRETCH ● OTHER

Time ☐ ☐ ☐ ☐ ☐ ☐

GLASSES OF WATER

STRESS 1 2 3 4 5 6 7 8 9 10

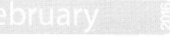

February

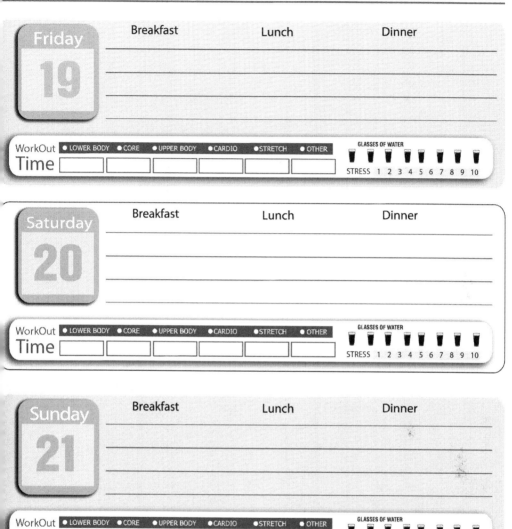

Friday 19

	Breakfast	Lunch	Dinner

WorkOut Time — ● LOWER BODY ● CORE ● UPPER BODY ● CARDIO ● STRETCH ● OTHER

GLASSES OF WATER
STRESS 1 2 3 4 5 6 7 8 9 10

Saturday 20

	Breakfast	Lunch	Dinner

WorkOut Time — ● LOWER BODY ● CORE ● UPPER BODY ● CARDIO ● STRETCH ● OTHER

GLASSES OF WATER
STRESS 1 2 3 4 5 6 7 8 9 10

Sunday 21

	Breakfast	Lunch	Dinner

WorkOut Time — ● LOWER BODY ● CORE ● UPPER BODY ● CARDIO ● STRETCH ● OTHER

GLASSES OF WATER
STRESS 1 2 3 4 5 6 7 8 9 10

Notes

Monday 22

Breakfast   Lunch   Dinner

WorkOut ● LOWER BODY ● CORE ● UPPER BODY ● CARDIO ● STRETCH ● OTHER
Time [ ] [ ] [ ] [ ] [ ] [ ]

GLASSES OF WATER
STRESS 1 2 3 4 5 6 7 8 9 10

Tuesday 23

Breakfast   Lunch   Dinner

WorkOut ● LOWER BODY ● CORE ● UPPER BODY ● CARDIO ● STRETCH ● OTHER
Time [ ] [ ] [ ] [ ] [ ] [ ]

GLASSES OF WATER
STRESS 1 2 3 4 5 6 7 8 9 10

Wednesday 24

Breakfast   Lunch   Dinner

WorkOut ● LOWER BODY ● CORE ● UPPER BODY ● CARDIO ● STRETCH ● OTHER
Time [ ] [ ] [ ] [ ] [ ] [ ]

GLASSES OF WATER
STRESS 1 2 3 4 5 6 7 8 9 10

Thursday 25

Breakfast   Lunch   Dinner

WorkOut ● LOWER BODY ● CORE ● UPPER BODY ● CARDIO ● STRETCH ● OTHER
Time [ ] [ ] [ ] [ ] [ ] [ ]

GLASSES OF WATER
STRESS 1 2 3 4 5 6 7 8 9 10

Friday 26

Breakfast	Lunch	Dinner

WorkOut Time: ● LOWER BODY ● CORE ● UPPER BODY ● CARDIO ● STRETCH ● OTHER

GLASSES OF WATER

STRESS 1 2 3 4 5 6 7 8 9 10

Saturday 27

Breakfast	Lunch	Dinner

WorkOut Time: ● LOWER BODY ● CORE ● UPPER BODY ● CARDIO ● STRETCH ● OTHER

GLASSES OF WATER

STRESS 1 2 3 4 5 6 7 8 9 10

Sunday 28

Breakfast	Lunch	Dinner

WorkOut Time: ● LOWER BODY ● CORE ● UPPER BODY ● CARDIO ● STRETCH ● OTHER

GLASSES OF WATER

STRESS 1 2 3 4 5 6 7 8 9 10

This Month's Measurements:

Waist
Neck
Biceps
Chest
Hips
Thighs

Month Progress Report

Current Weight:

Notes:

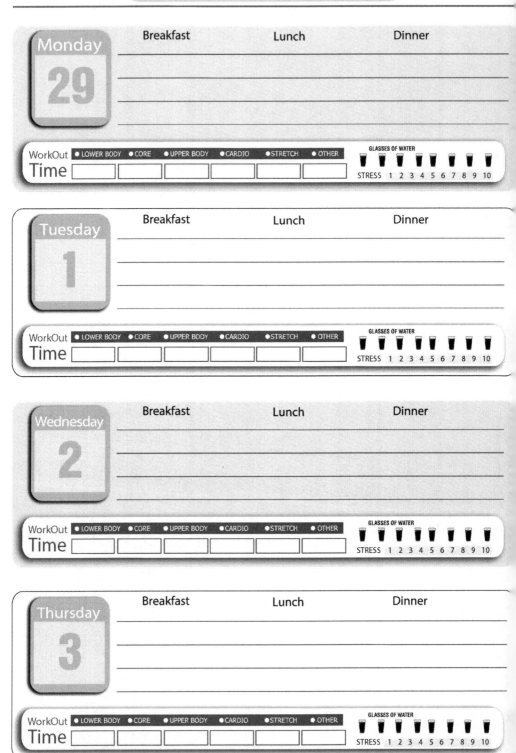

Monday 29

Breakfast   Lunch   Dinner

WorkOut   ● LOWER BODY   ● CORE   ● UPPER BODY   ● CARDIO   ● STRETCH   ● OTHER

Time

GLASSES OF WATER

STRESS 1 2 3 4 5 6 7 8 9 10

Tuesday 1

Breakfast   Lunch   Dinner

WorkOut   ● LOWER BODY   ● CORE   ● UPPER BODY   ● CARDIO   ● STRETCH   ● OTHER

Time

GLASSES OF WATER

STRESS 1 2 3 4 5 6 7 8 9 10

Wednesday 2

Breakfast   Lunch   Dinner

WorkOut   ● LOWER BODY   ● CORE   ● UPPER BODY   ● CARDIO   ● STRETCH   ● OTHER

Time

GLASSES OF WATER

STRESS 1 2 3 4 5 6 7 8 9 10

Thursday 3

Breakfast   Lunch   Dinner

WorkOut   ● LOWER BODY   ● CORE   ● UPPER BODY   ● CARDIO   ● STRETCH   ● OTHER

Time

GLASSES OF WATER

STRESS 1 2 3 4 5 6 7 8 9 10

March

Friday 4

Breakfast   Lunch   Dinner

WorkOut Time   ● LOWER BODY   ● CORE   ● UPPER BODY   ● CARDIO   ● STRETCH   ● OTHER

GLASSES OF WATER

STRESS   1   2   3   4   5   6   7   8   9   10

Saturday 5

Breakfast   Lunch   Dinner

WorkOut Time   ● LOWER BODY   ● CORE   ● UPPER BODY   ● CARDIO   ● STRETCH   ● OTHER

GLASSES OF WATER

STRESS   1   2   3   4   5   6   7   8   9   10

Sunday 6

Breakfast   Lunch   Dinner

WorkOut Time   ● LOWER BODY   ● CORE   ● UPPER BODY   ● CARDIO   ● STRETCH   ● OTHER

GLASSES OF WATER

STRESS   1   2   3   4   5   6   7   8   9   10

Notes

Monday 7

	Breakfast	Lunch	Dinner

WorkOut ● LOWER BODY ● CORE ● UPPER BODY ● CARDIO ● STRETCH ● OTHER

Time

GLASSES OF WATER

STRESS 1 2 3 4 5 6 7 8 9 10

Tuesday 8

	Breakfast	Lunch	Dinner

WorkOut ● LOWER BODY ● CORE ● UPPER BODY ● CARDIO ● STRETCH ● OTHER

Time

GLASSES OF WATER

STRESS 1 2 3 4 5 6 7 8 9 10

Wednesday 9

	Breakfast	Lunch	Dinner

WorkOut ● LOWER BODY ● CORE ● UPPER BODY ● CARDIO ● STRETCH ● OTHER

Time

GLASSES OF WATER

STRESS 1 2 3 4 5 6 7 8 9 10

Thursday 10

	Breakfast	Lunch	Dinner

WorkOut ● LOWER BODY ● CORE ● UPPER BODY ● CARDIO ● STRETCH ● OTHER

Time

GLASSES OF WATER

STRESS 1 2 3 4 5 6 7 8 9 10

Friday 11

Breakfast | Lunch | Dinner

WorkOut: ● LOWER BODY ● CORE ● UPPER BODY ● CARDIO ● STRETCH ● OTHER
Time: [ ] [ ] [ ] [ ] [ ] [ ]
GLASSES OF WATER
STRESS 1 2 3 4 5 6 7 8 9 10

Saturday 12

Breakfast | Lunch | Dinner

WorkOut: ● LOWER BODY ● CORE ● UPPER BODY ● CARDIO ● STRETCH ● OTHER
Time: [ ] [ ] [ ] [ ] [ ] [ ]
GLASSES OF WATER
STRESS 1 2 3 4 5 6 7 8 9 10

Sunday 13

Breakfast | Lunch | Dinner

WorkOut: ● LOWER BODY ● CORE ● UPPER BODY ● CARDIO ● STRETCH ● OTHER
Time: [ ] [ ] [ ] [ ] [ ] [ ]
GLASSES OF WATER
STRESS 1 2 3 4 5 6 7 8 9 10

Notes

Monday 14

	Breakfast	Lunch	Dinner

WorkOut Time: ● LOWER BODY ● CORE ● UPPER BODY ● CARDIO ● STRETCH ● OTHER

GLASSES OF WATER
STRESS 1 2 3 4 5 6 7 8 9 10

Tuesday 15

	Breakfast	Lunch	Dinner

WorkOut Time: ● LOWER BODY ● CORE ● UPPER BODY ● CARDIO ● STRETCH ● OTHER

GLASSES OF WATER
STRESS 1 2 3 4 5 6 7 8 9 10

Wednesday 16

	Breakfast	Lunch	Dinner

WorkOut Time: ● LOWER BODY ● CORE ● UPPER BODY ● CARDIO ● STRETCH ● OTHER

GLASSES OF WATER
STRESS 1 2 3 4 5 6 7 8 9 10

Thursday 17

	Breakfast	Lunch	Dinner

WorkOut Time: ● LOWER BODY ● CORE ● UPPER BODY ● CARDIO ● STRETCH ● OTHER

GLASSES OF WATER
STRESS 1 2 3 4 5 6 7 8 9 10

Friday 18

Breakfast	Lunch	Dinner

WorkOut Time
● LOWER BODY ● CORE ● UPPER BODY ● CARDIO ● STRETCH ● OTHER

GLASSES OF WATER
STRESS 1 2 3 4 5 6 7 8 9 10

Saturday 19

Breakfast	Lunch	Dinner

WorkOut Time
● LOWER BODY ● CORE ● UPPER BODY ● CARDIO ● STRETCH ● OTHER

GLASSES OF WATER
STRESS 1 2 3 4 5 6 7 8 9 10

Sunday 20

Breakfast	Lunch	Dinner

WorkOut Time
● LOWER BODY ● CORE ● UPPER BODY ● CARDIO ● STRETCH ● OTHER

GLASSES OF WATER
STRESS 1 2 3 4 5 6 7 8 9 10

Notes

March 2016

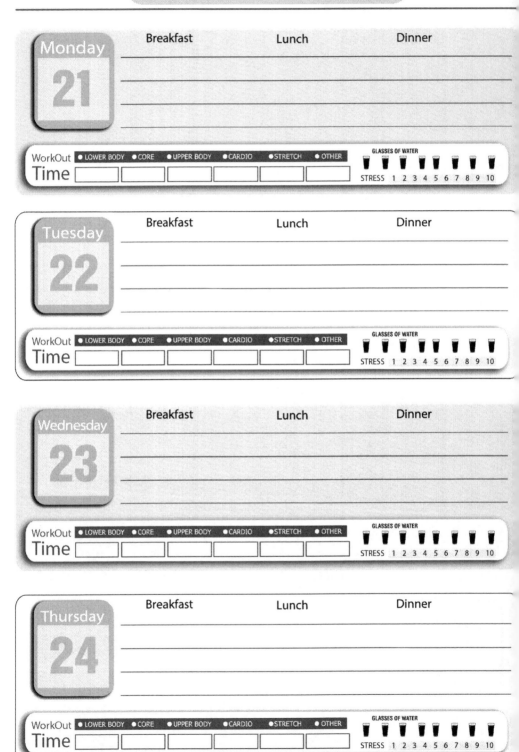

Monday 21

Breakfast   Lunch   Dinner

WorkOut ● LOWER BODY ● CORE ● UPPER BODY ● CARDIO ● STRETCH ● OTHER
Time

GLASSES OF WATER
STRESS 1 2 3 4 5 6 7 8 9 10

Tuesday 22

Breakfast   Lunch   Dinner

WorkOut ● LOWER BODY ● CORE ● UPPER BODY ● CARDIO ● STRETCH ● OTHER
Time

GLASSES OF WATER
STRESS 1 2 3 4 5 6 7 8 9 10

Wednesday 23

Breakfast   Lunch   Dinner

WorkOut ● LOWER BODY ● CORE ● UPPER BODY ● CARDIO ● STRETCH ● OTHER
Time

GLASSES OF WATER
STRESS 1 2 3 4 5 6 7 8 9 10

Thursday 24

Breakfast   Lunch   Dinner

WorkOut ● LOWER BODY ● CORE ● UPPER BODY ● CARDIO ● STRETCH ● OTHER
Time

GLASSES OF WATER
STRESS 1 2 3 4 5 6 7 8 9 10

Friday 25

	Breakfast	Lunch	Dinner

WorkOut
Time
● LOWER BODY ● CORE ● UPPER BODY ● CARDIO ● STRETCH ● OTHER

GLASSES OF WATER
STRESS 1 2 3 4 5 6 7 8 9 10

Saturday 26

	Breakfast	Lunch	Dinner

WorkOut
Time
● LOWER BODY ● CORE ● UPPER BODY ● CARDIO ● STRETCH ● OTHER

GLASSES OF WATER
STRESS 1 2 3 4 5 6 7 8 9 10

Sunday 27

	Breakfast	Lunch	Dinner

WorkOut
Time
● LOWER BODY ● CORE ● UPPER BODY ● CARDIO ● STRETCH ● OTHER

GLASSES OF WATER
STRESS 1 2 3 4 5 6 7 8 9 10

Notes

Monday 28

	Breakfast	Lunch	Dinner

WorkOut ● LOWER BODY ● CORE ● UPPER BODY ● CARDIO ● STRETCH ● OTHER
Time

GLASSES OF WATER
STRESS 1 2 3 4 5 6 7 8 9 10

Tuesday 29

	Breakfast	Lunch	Dinner

WorkOut ● LOWER BODY ● CORE ● UPPER BODY ● CARDIO ● STRETCH ● OTHER
Time

GLASSES OF WATER
STRESS 1 2 3 4 5 6 7 8 9 10

Wednesday 30

	Breakfast	Lunch	Dinner

WorkOut ● LOWER BODY ● CORE ● UPPER BODY ● CARDIO ● STRETCH ● OTHER
Time

GLASSES OF WATER
STRESS 1 2 3 4 5 6 7 8 9 10

Thursday 31

	Breakfast	Lunch	Dinner

WorkOut ● LOWER BODY ● CORE ● UPPER BODY ● CARDIO ● STRETCH ● OTHER
Time

GLASSES OF WATER
STRESS 1 2 3 4 5 6 7 8 9 10

Friday 1

Breakfast	Lunch	Dinner

WorkOut Time
● LOWER BODY ● CORE ● UPPER BODY ● CARDIO ● STRETCH ● OTHER

GLASSES OF WATER
STRESS 1 2 3 4 5 6 7 8 9 10

Saturday 2

Breakfast	Lunch	Dinner

WorkOut Time
● LOWER BODY ● CORE ● UPPER BODY ● CARDIO ● STRETCH ● OTHER

GLASSES OF WATER
STRESS 1 2 3 4 5 6 7 8 9 10

Sunday 3

Breakfast	Lunch	Dinner

WorkOut Time
● LOWER BODY ● CORE ● UPPER BODY ● CARDIO ● STRETCH ● OTHER

GLASSES OF WATER
STRESS 1 2 3 4 5 6 7 8 9 10

This Month's Measurements:

Waist
Neck
Biceps
Chest
Hips
Thighs

Month Progress Report

Current Weight:

Notes:

April 2016

Monday 4

Breakfast	Lunch	Dinner

WorkOut ● LOWER BODY ● CORE ● UPPER BODY ● CARDIO ● STRETCH ● OTHER
Time [ ] [ ] [ ] [ ] [ ] [ ]

GLASSES OF WATER
STRESS 1 2 3 4 5 6 7 8 9 10

Tuesday 5

Breakfast	Lunch	Dinner

WorkOut ● LOWER BODY ● CORE ● UPPER BODY ● CARDIO ● STRETCH ● OTHER
Time [ ] [ ] [ ] [ ] [ ] [ ]

GLASSES OF WATER
STRESS 1 2 3 4 5 6 7 8 9 10

Wednesday 6

Breakfast	Lunch	Dinner

WorkOut ● LOWER BODY ● CORE ● UPPER BODY ● CARDIO ● STRETCH ● OTHER
Time [ ] [ ] [ ] [ ] [ ] [ ]

GLASSES OF WATER
STRESS 1 2 3 4 5 6 7 8 9 10

Thursday 7

Breakfast	Lunch	Dinner

WorkOut ● LOWER BODY ● CORE ● UPPER BODY ● CARDIO ● STRETCH ● OTHER
Time [ ] [ ] [ ] [ ] [ ] [ ]

GLASSES OF WATER
STRESS 1 2 3 4 5 6 7 8 9 10

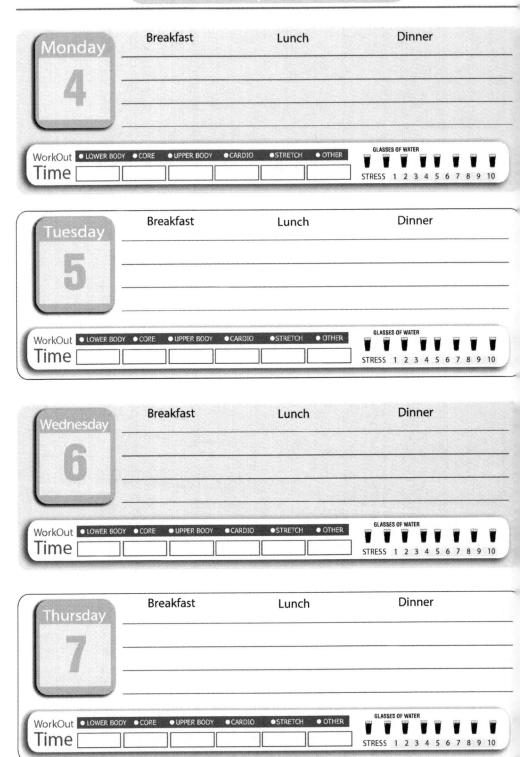

Friday 8

Breakfast	Lunch	Dinner

WorkOut Time ● LOWER BODY ● CORE ● UPPER BODY ● CARDIO ● STRETCH ● OTHER

GLASSES OF WATER
STRESS 1 2 3 4 5 6 7 8 9 10

Saturday 9

Breakfast	Lunch	Dinner

WorkOut Time ● LOWER BODY ● CORE ● UPPER BODY ● CARDIO ● STRETCH ● OTHER

GLASSES OF WATER
STRESS 1 2 3 4 5 6 7 8 9 10

Sunday 10

Breakfast	Lunch	Dinner

WorkOut Time ● LOWER BODY ● CORE ● UPPER BODY ● CARDIO ● STRETCH ● OTHER

GLASSES OF WATER
STRESS 1 2 3 4 5 6 7 8 9 10

Notes

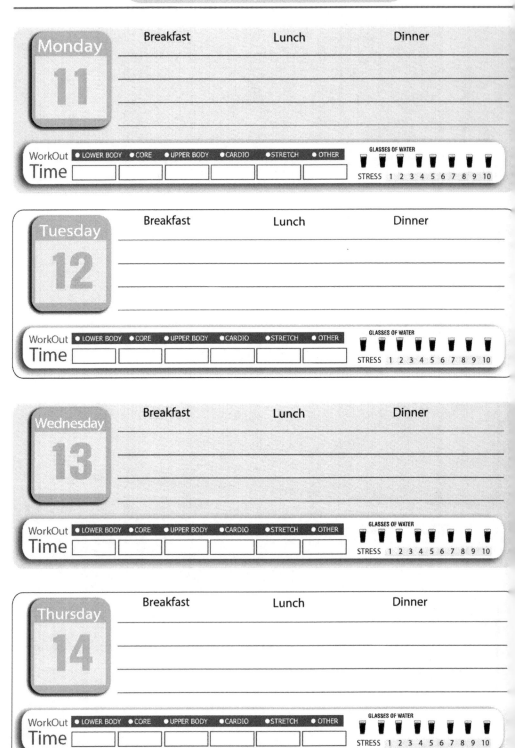

Monday 11

Breakfast	Lunch	Dinner

WorkOut ● LOWER BODY ● CORE ● UPPER BODY ● CARDIO ● STRETCH ● OTHER
Time

GLASSES OF WATER
STRESS 1 2 3 4 5 6 7 8 9 10

Tuesday 12

Breakfast	Lunch	Dinner

WorkOut ● LOWER BODY ● CORE ● UPPER BODY ● CARDIO ● STRETCH ● OTHER
Time

GLASSES OF WATER
STRESS 1 2 3 4 5 6 7 8 9 10

Wednesday 13

Breakfast	Lunch	Dinner

WorkOut ● LOWER BODY ● CORE ● UPPER BODY ● CARDIO ● STRETCH ● OTHER
Time

GLASSES OF WATER
STRESS 1 2 3 4 5 6 7 8 9 10

Thursday 14

Breakfast	Lunch	Dinner

WorkOut ● LOWER BODY ● CORE ● UPPER BODY ● CARDIO ● STRETCH ● OTHER
Time

GLASSES OF WATER
STRESS 1 2 3 4 5 6 7 8 9 10

Friday 15

Breakfast   Lunch   Dinner

WorkOut Time ● LOWER BODY ● CORE ● UPPER BODY ● CARDIO ● STRETCH ● OTHER

GLASSES OF WATER
STRESS 1 2 3 4 5 6 7 8 9 10

Saturday 16

Breakfast   Lunch   Dinner

WorkOut Time ● LOWER BODY ● CORE ● UPPER BODY ● CARDIO ● STRETCH ● OTHER

GLASSES OF WATER
STRESS 1 2 3 4 5 6 7 8 9 10

Sunday 17

Breakfast   Lunch   Dinner

WorkOut Time ● LOWER BODY ● CORE ● UPPER BODY ● CARDIO ● STRETCH ● OTHER

GLASSES OF WATER
STRESS 1 2 3 4 5 6 7 8 9 10

Notes

Monday 18

	Breakfast	Lunch	Dinner

WorkOut ● LOWER BODY ● CORE ● UPPER BODY ● CARDIO ● STRETCH ● OTHER

Time ☐ ☐ ☐ ☐ ☐ ☐

GLASSES OF WATER

STRESS 1 2 3 4 5 6 7 8 9 10

Tuesday 19

	Breakfast	Lunch	Dinner

WorkOut ● LOWER BODY ● CORE ● UPPER BODY ● CARDIO ● STRETCH ● OTHER

Time ☐ ☐ ☐ ☐ ☐ ☐

GLASSES OF WATER

STRESS 1 2 3 4 5 6 7 8 9 10

Wednesday 20

	Breakfast	Lunch	Dinner

WorkOut ● LOWER BODY ● CORE ● UPPER BODY ● CARDIO ● STRETCH ● OTHER

Time ☐ ☐ ☐ ☐ ☐ ☐

GLASSES OF WATER

STRESS 1 2 3 4 5 6 7 8 9 10

Thursday 21

	Breakfast	Lunch	Dinner

WorkOut ● LOWER BODY ● CORE ● UPPER BODY ● CARDIO ● STRETCH ● OTHER

Time ☐ ☐ ☐ ☐ ☐ ☐

GLASSES OF WATER

STRESS 1 2 3 4 5 6 7 8 9 10

Friday 22

Breakfast	Lunch	Dinner

WorkOut ● LOWER BODY ● CORE ● UPPER BODY ● CARDIO ● STRETCH ● OTHER

Time

GLASSES OF WATER

STRESS 1 2 3 4 5 6 7 8 9 10

Saturday 23

Breakfast	Lunch	Dinner

WorkOut ● LOWER BODY ● CORE ● UPPER BODY ● CARDIO ● STRETCH ● OTHER

Time

GLASSES OF WATER

STRESS 1 2 3 4 5 6 7 8 9 10

Sunday 24

Breakfast	Lunch	Dinner

WorkOut ● LOWER BODY ● CORE ● UPPER BODY ● CARDIO ● STRETCH ● OTHER

Time

GLASSES OF WATER

STRESS 1 2 3 4 5 6 7 8 9 10

Notes

April 2016

Monday 25

	Breakfast	Lunch	Dinner

WorkOut Time — ● LOWER BODY ● CORE ● UPPER BODY ● CARDIO ● STRETCH ● OTHER

GLASSES OF WATER
STRESS 1 2 3 4 5 6 7 8 9 10

Tuesday 26

	Breakfast	Lunch	Dinner

WorkOut Time — ● LOWER BODY ● CORE ● UPPER BODY ● CARDIO ● STRETCH ● OTHER

GLASSES OF WATER
STRESS 1 2 3 4 5 6 7 8 9 10

Wednesday 27

	Breakfast	Lunch	Dinner

WorkOut Time — ● LOWER BODY ● CORE ● UPPER BODY ● CARDIO ● STRETCH ● OTHER

GLASSES OF WATER
STRESS 1 2 3 4 5 6 7 8 9 10

Thursday 28

	Breakfast	Lunch	Dinner

WorkOut Time — ● LOWER BODY ● CORE ● UPPER BODY ● CARDIO ● STRETCH ● OTHER

GLASSES OF WATER
STRESS 1 2 3 4 5 6 7 8 9 10

Friday
29

Breakfast	Lunch	Dinner

WorkOut — ● LOWER BODY ● CORE ● UPPER BODY ● CARDIO ● STRETCH ● OTHER
Time [ ] [ ] [ ] [ ] [ ] [ ]

GLASSES OF WATER
STRESS 1 2 3 4 5 6 7 8 9 10

Saturday
30

Breakfast	Lunch	Dinner

WorkOut — ● LOWER BODY ● CORE ● UPPER BODY ● CARDIO ● STRETCH ● OTHER
Time [ ] [ ] [ ] [ ] [ ] [ ]

GLASSES OF WATER
STRESS 1 2 3 4 5 6 7 8 9 10

Sunday
1

Breakfast	Lunch	Dinner

WorkOut — ● LOWER BODY ● CORE ● UPPER BODY ● CARDIO ● STRETCH ● OTHER
Time [ ] [ ] [ ] [ ] [ ] [ ]

GLASSES OF WATER
STRESS 1 2 3 4 5 6 7 8 9 10

This Month's Measurements:

Waist
Neck
Biceps
Chest
Hips
Thighs

Month Progress Report

Current Weight:

Notes:

Monday 2

	Breakfast	Lunch	Dinner

WorkOut Time | ● LOWER BODY | ● CORE | ● UPPER BODY | ● CARDIO | ● STRETCH | ● OTHER

GLASSES OF WATER

STRESS 1 2 3 4 5 6 7 8 9 10

Tuesday 3

	Breakfast	Lunch	Dinner

WorkOut Time | ● LOWER BODY | ● CORE | ● UPPER BODY | ● CARDIO | ● STRETCH | ● OTHER

GLASSES OF WATER

STRESS 1 2 3 4 5 6 7 8 9 10

Wednesday 4

	Breakfast	Lunch	Dinner

WorkOut Time | ● LOWER BODY | ● CORE | ● UPPER BODY | ● CARDIO | ● STRETCH | ● OTHER

GLASSES OF WATER

STRESS 1 2 3 4 5 6 7 8 9 10

Thursday 5

	Breakfast	Lunch	Dinner

WorkOut Time | ● LOWER BODY | ● CORE | ● UPPER BODY | ● CARDIO | ● STRETCH | ● OTHER

GLASSES OF WATER

STRESS 1 2 3 4 5 6 7 8 9 10

May 2016

Friday 6

Breakfast _____
Lunch _____
Dinner _____

WorkOut Time
● LOWER BODY ● CORE ● UPPER BODY ● CARDIO ● STRETCH ● OTHER

GLASSES OF WATER
STRESS 1 2 3 4 5 6 7 8 9 10

Saturday 7

Breakfast _____
Lunch _____
Dinner _____

WorkOut Time
● LOWER BODY ● CORE ● UPPER BODY ● CARDIO ● STRETCH ● OTHER

GLASSES OF WATER
STRESS 1 2 3 4 5 6 7 8 9 10

Sunday 8

Breakfast _____
Lunch _____
Dinner _____

WorkOut Time
● LOWER BODY ● CORE ● UPPER BODY ● CARDIO ● STRETCH ● OTHER

GLASSES OF WATER
STRESS 1 2 3 4 5 6 7 8 9 10

Notes

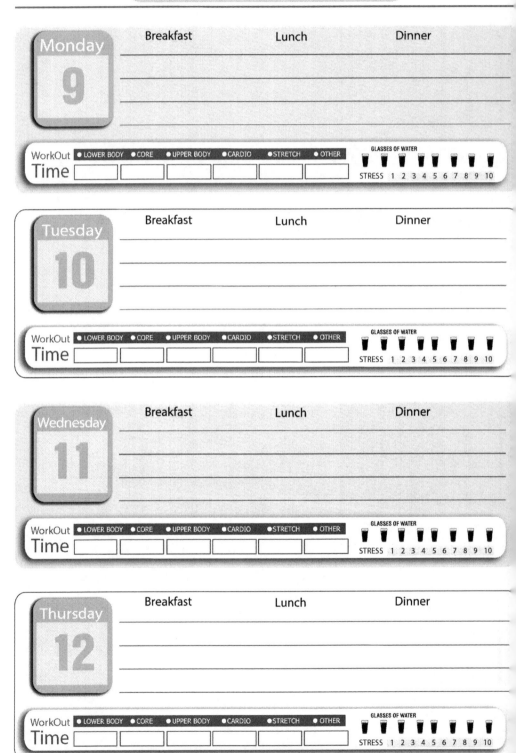

May 2016

Monday 9

Breakfast	Lunch	Dinner

WorkOut ● LOWER BODY ● CORE ● UPPER BODY ● CARDIO ● STRETCH ● OTHER
Time

GLASSES OF WATER
STRESS 1 2 3 4 5 6 7 8 9 10

Tuesday 10

Breakfast	Lunch	Dinner

WorkOut ● LOWER BODY ● CORE ● UPPER BODY ● CARDIO ● STRETCH ● OTHER
Time

GLASSES OF WATER
STRESS 1 2 3 4 5 6 7 8 9 10

Wednesday 11

Breakfast	Lunch	Dinner

WorkOut ● LOWER BODY ● CORE ● UPPER BODY ● CARDIO ● STRETCH ● OTHER
Time

GLASSES OF WATER
STRESS 1 2 3 4 5 6 7 8 9 10

Thursday 12

Breakfast	Lunch	Dinner

WorkOut ● LOWER BODY ● CORE ● UPPER BODY ● CARDIO ● STRETCH ● OTHER
Time

GLASSES OF WATER
STRESS 1 2 3 4 5 6 7 8 9 10

May

2016

Friday 13

Breakfast | Lunch | Dinner

WorkOut Time
● LOWER BODY ● CORE ● UPPER BODY ● CARDIO ● STRETCH ● OTHER

GLASSES OF WATER
STRESS 1 2 3 4 5 6 7 8 9 10

Saturday 14

Breakfast | Lunch | Dinner

WorkOut Time
● LOWER BODY ● CORE ● UPPER BODY ● CARDIO ● STRETCH ● OTHER

GLASSES OF WATER
STRESS 1 2 3 4 5 6 7 8 9 10

Sunday 15

Breakfast | Lunch | Dinner

WorkOut Time
● LOWER BODY ● CORE ● UPPER BODY ● CARDIO ● STRETCH ● OTHER

GLASSES OF WATER
STRESS 1 2 3 4 5 6 7 8 9 10

Notes

Monday 16

	Breakfast	Lunch	Dinner

WorkOut Time — ● LOWER BODY ● CORE ● UPPER BODY ● CARDIO ● STRETCH ● OTHER

GLASSES OF WATER

STRESS 1 2 3 4 5 6 7 8 9 10

Tuesday 17

	Breakfast	Lunch	Dinner

WorkOut Time — ● LOWER BODY ● CORE ● UPPER BODY ● CARDIO ● STRETCH ● OTHER

GLASSES OF WATER

STRESS 1 2 3 4 5 6 7 8 9 10

Wednesday 18

	Breakfast	Lunch	Dinner

WorkOut Time — ● LOWER BODY ● CORE ● UPPER BODY ● CARDIO ● STRETCH ● OTHER

GLASSES OF WATER

STRESS 1 2 3 4 5 6 7 8 9 10

Thursday 19

	Breakfast	Lunch	Dinner

WorkOut Time — ● LOWER BODY ● CORE ● UPPER BODY ● CARDIO ● STRETCH ● OTHER

GLASSES OF WATER

STRESS 1 2 3 4 5 6 7 8 9 10

Friday 20

Breakfast	Lunch	Dinner

WorkOut Time: ● LOWER BODY ● CORE ● UPPER BODY ● CARDIO ● STRETCH ● OTHER

GLASSES OF WATER
STRESS 1 2 3 4 5 6 7 8 9 10

Saturday 21

Breakfast	Lunch	Dinner

WorkOut Time: ● LOWER BODY ● CORE ● UPPER BODY ● CARDIO ● STRETCH ● OTHER

GLASSES OF WATER
STRESS 1 2 3 4 5 6 7 8 9 10

Sunday 22

Breakfast	Lunch	Dinner

WorkOut Time: ● LOWER BODY ● CORE ● UPPER BODY ● CARDIO ● STRETCH ● OTHER

GLASSES OF WATER
STRESS 1 2 3 4 5 6 7 8 9 10

Notes

May 2016

Monday 23

Breakfast   Lunch   Dinner

WorkOut   ● LOWER BODY   ● CORE   ● UPPER BODY   ● CARDIO   ● STRETCH   ● OTHER

Time

GLASSES OF WATER

STRESS   1   2   3   4   5   6   7   8   9   10

Tuesday 24

Breakfast   Lunch   Dinner

WorkOut   ● LOWER BODY   ● CORE   ● UPPER BODY   ● CARDIO   ● STRETCH   ● OTHER

Time

GLASSES OF WATER

STRESS   1   2   3   4   5   6   7   8   9   10

Wednesday 25

Breakfast   Lunch   Dinner

WorkOut   ● LOWER BODY   ● CORE   ● UPPER BODY   ● CARDIO   ● STRETCH   ● OTHER

Time

GLASSES OF WATER

STRESS   1   2   3   4   5   6   7   8   9   10

Thursday 26

Breakfast   Lunch   Dinner

WorkOut   ● LOWER BODY   ● CORE   ● UPPER BODY   ● CARDIO   ● STRETCH   ● OTHER

Time

GLASSES OF WATER

STRESS   1   2   3   4   5   6   7   8   9   10

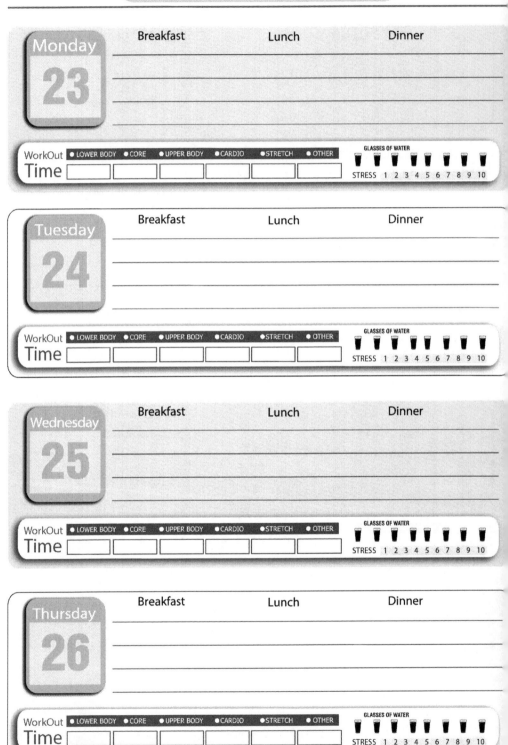

Friday 27

Breakfast	Lunch	Dinner

WorkOut ● LOWER BODY ● CORE ● UPPER BODY ● CARDIO ● STRETCH ● OTHER

Time [ ] [ ] [ ] [ ] [ ] [ ]

GLASSES OF WATER

STRESS 1 2 3 4 5 6 7 8 9 10

Saturday 28

Breakfast	Lunch	Dinner

WorkOut ● LOWER BODY ● CORE ● UPPER BODY ● CARDIO ● STRETCH ● OTHER

Time [ ] [ ] [ ] [ ] [ ] [ ]

GLASSES OF WATER

STRESS 1 2 3 4 5 6 7 8 9 10

Sunday 29

Breakfast	Lunch	Dinner

WorkOut ● LOWER BODY ● CORE ● UPPER BODY ● CARDIO ● STRETCH ● OTHER

Time [ ] [ ] [ ] [ ] [ ] [ ]

GLASSES OF WATER

STRESS 1 2 3 4 5 6 7 8 9 10

This Month's Measurements:

Waist
Neck
Biceps
Chest
Hips
Thighs

Month Progress Report

Current Weight:

Notes:

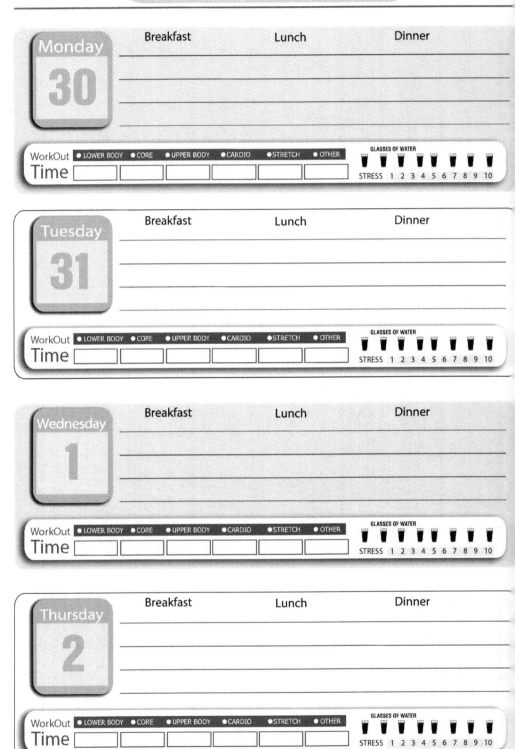

Monday 30

Breakfast | Lunch | Dinner

WorkOut — ● LOWER BODY ● CORE ● UPPER BODY ● CARDIO ● STRETCH ● OTHER
Time

GLASSES OF WATER
STRESS 1 2 3 4 5 6 7 8 9 10

Tuesday 31

Breakfast | Lunch | Dinner

WorkOut — ● LOWER BODY ● CORE ● UPPER BODY ● CARDIO ● STRETCH ● OTHER
Time

GLASSES OF WATER
STRESS 1 2 3 4 5 6 7 8 9 10

Wednesday 1

Breakfast | Lunch | Dinner

WorkOut — ● LOWER BODY ● CORE ● UPPER BODY ● CARDIO ● STRETCH ● OTHER
Time

GLASSES OF WATER
STRESS 1 2 3 4 5 6 7 8 9 10

Thursday 2

Breakfast | Lunch | Dinner

WorkOut — ● LOWER BODY ● CORE ● UPPER BODY ● CARDIO ● STRETCH ● OTHER
Time

GLASSES OF WATER
STRESS 1 2 3 4 5 6 7 8 9 10

June

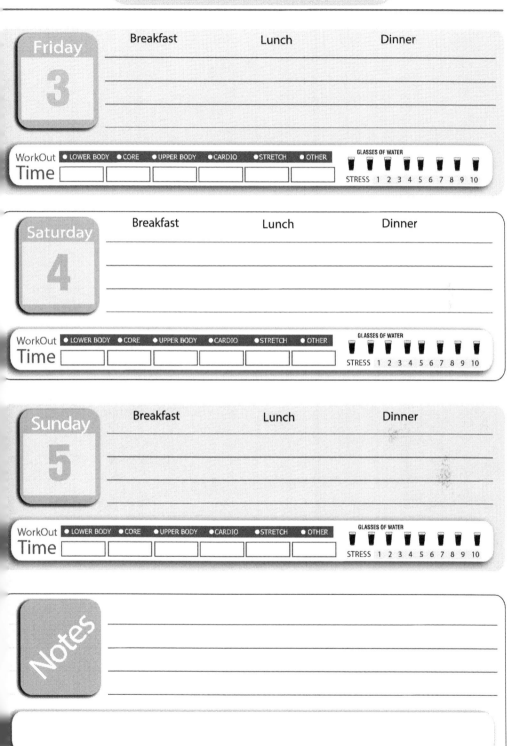

Friday
3

Breakfast   Lunch   Dinner

WorkOut ●LOWER BODY ●CORE ●UPPER BODY ●CARDIO ●STRETCH ●OTHER

Time

GLASSES OF WATER

STRESS 1 2 3 4 5 6 7 8 9 10

Saturday
4

Breakfast   Lunch   Dinner

WorkOut ●LOWER BODY ●CORE ●UPPER BODY ●CARDIO ●STRETCH ●OTHER

Time

GLASSES OF WATER

STRESS 1 2 3 4 5 6 7 8 9 10

Sunday
5

Breakfast   Lunch   Dinner

WorkOut ●LOWER BODY ●CORE ●UPPER BODY ●CARDIO ●STRETCH ●OTHER

Time

GLASSES OF WATER

STRESS 1 2 3 4 5 6 7 8 9 10

Notes

Monday 6

Breakfast	Lunch	Dinner

WorkOut ● LOWER BODY ● CORE ● UPPER BODY ● CARDIO ● STRETCH ● OTHER
Time [ ] [ ] [ ] [ ] [ ] [ ]

GLASSES OF WATER
STRESS 1 2 3 4 5 6 7 8 9 10

Tuesday 7

Breakfast	Lunch	Dinner

WorkOut ● LOWER BODY ● CORE ● UPPER BODY ● CARDIO ● STRETCH ● OTHER
Time [ ] [ ] [ ] [ ] [ ] [ ]

GLASSES OF WATER
STRESS 1 2 3 4 5 6 7 8 9 10

Wednesday 8

Breakfast	Lunch	Dinner

WorkOut ● LOWER BODY ● CORE ● UPPER BODY ● CARDIO ● STRETCH ● OTHER
Time [ ] [ ] [ ] [ ] [ ] [ ]

GLASSES OF WATER
STRESS 1 2 3 4 5 6 7 8 9 10

Thursday 9

Breakfast	Lunch	Dinner

WorkOut ● LOWER BODY ● CORE ● UPPER BODY ● CARDIO ● STRETCH ● OTHER
Time [ ] [ ] [ ] [ ] [ ] [ ]

GLASSES OF WATER
STRESS 1 2 3 4 5 6 7 8 9 10

Friday
10

Breakfast   Lunch   Dinner

WorkOut ● LOWER BODY ● CORE ● UPPER BODY ● CARDIO ● STRETCH ● OTHER

Time

GLASSES OF WATER

STRESS 1 2 3 4 5 6 7 8 9 10

Saturday
11

Breakfast   Lunch   Dinner

WorkOut ● LOWER BODY ● CORE ● UPPER BODY ● CARDIO ● STRETCH ● OTHER

Time

GLASSES OF WATER

STRESS 1 2 3 4 5 6 7 8 9 10

Sunday
12

Breakfast   Lunch   Dinner

WorkOut ● LOWER BODY ● CORE ● UPPER BODY ● CARDIO ● STRETCH ● OTHER

Time

GLASSES OF WATER

STRESS 1 2 3 4 5 6 7 8 9 10

Notes

Monday 13

Breakfast	Lunch	Dinner

WorkOut ● LOWER BODY ● CORE ● UPPER BODY ● CARDIO ● STRETCH ● OTHER
Time

GLASSES OF WATER
STRESS 1 2 3 4 5 6 7 8 9 10

Tuesday 14

Breakfast	Lunch	Dinner

WorkOut ● LOWER BODY ● CORE ● UPPER BODY ● CARDIO ● STRETCH ● OTHER
Time

GLASSES OF WATER
STRESS 1 2 3 4 5 6 7 8 9 10

Wednesday 15

Breakfast	Lunch	Dinner

WorkOut ● LOWER BODY ● CORE ● UPPER BODY ● CARDIO ● STRETCH ● OTHER
Time

GLASSES OF WATER
STRESS 1 2 3 4 5 6 7 8 9 10

Thursday 16

Breakfast	Lunch	Dinner

WorkOut ● LOWER BODY ● CORE ● UPPER BODY ● CARDIO ● STRETCH ● OTHER
Time

GLASSES OF WATER
STRESS 1 2 3 4 5 6 7 8 9 10

June

Friday 17

	Breakfast	Lunch	Dinner

WorkOut Time | ● LOWER BODY | ● CORE | ● UPPER BODY | ● CARDIO | ● STRETCH | ● OTHER

GLASSES OF WATER

STRESS 1 2 3 4 5 6 7 8 9 10

Saturday 18

	Breakfast	Lunch	Dinner

WorkOut Time | ● LOWER BODY | ● CORE | ● UPPER BODY | ● CARDIO | ● STRETCH | ● OTHER

GLASSES OF WATER

STRESS 1 2 3 4 5 6 7 8 9 10

Sunday 19

	Breakfast	Lunch	Dinner

WorkOut Time | ● LOWER BODY | ● CORE | ● UPPER BODY | ● CARDIO | ● STRETCH | ● OTHER

GLASSES OF WATER

STRESS 1 2 3 4 5 6 7 8 9 10

Notes

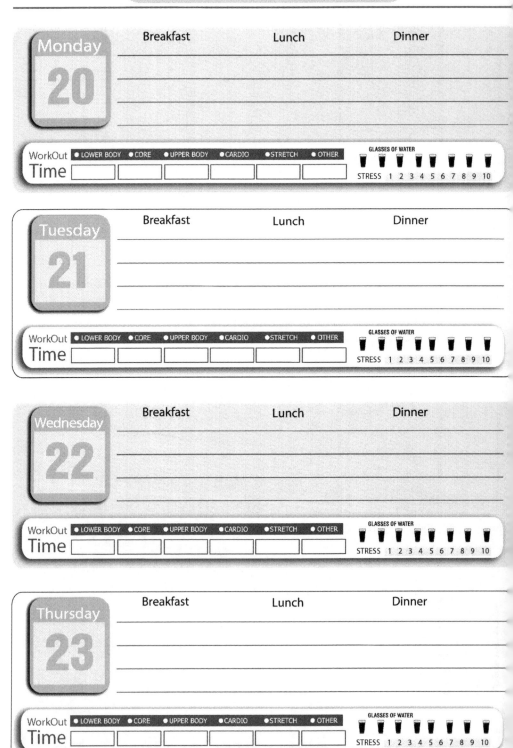

June 2016

Monday 20

Breakfast

Lunch

Dinner

WorkOut Time — LOWER BODY · CORE · UPPER BODY · CARDIO · STRETCH · OTHER

GLASSES OF WATER
STRESS 1 2 3 4 5 6 7 8 9 10

Tuesday 21

Breakfast

Lunch

Dinner

WorkOut Time — LOWER BODY · CORE · UPPER BODY · CARDIO · STRETCH · OTHER

GLASSES OF WATER
STRESS 1 2 3 4 5 6 7 8 9 10

Wednesday 22

Breakfast

Lunch

Dinner

WorkOut Time — LOWER BODY · CORE · UPPER BODY · CARDIO · STRETCH · OTHER

GLASSES OF WATER
STRESS 1 2 3 4 5 6 7 8 9 10

Thursday 23

Breakfast

Lunch

Dinner

WorkOut Time — LOWER BODY · CORE · UPPER BODY · CARDIO · STRETCH · OTHER

GLASSES OF WATER
STRESS 1 2 3 4 5 6 7 8 9 10

June

Friday 24

Breakfast	Lunch	Dinner

WorkOut Time ● LOWER BODY ● CORE ● UPPER BODY ● CARDIO ● STRETCH ● OTHER

GLASSES OF WATER

STRESS 1 2 3 4 5 6 7 8 9 10

Saturday 25

Breakfast	Lunch	Dinner

WorkOut Time ● LOWER BODY ● CORE ● UPPER BODY ● CARDIO ● STRETCH ● OTHER

GLASSES OF WATER

STRESS 1 2 3 4 5 6 7 8 9 10

Sunday 26

Breakfast	Lunch	Dinner

WorkOut Time ● LOWER BODY ● CORE ● UPPER BODY ● CARDIO ● STRETCH ● OTHER

GLASSES OF WATER

STRESS 1 2 3 4 5 6 7 8 9 10

Notes

June 2016

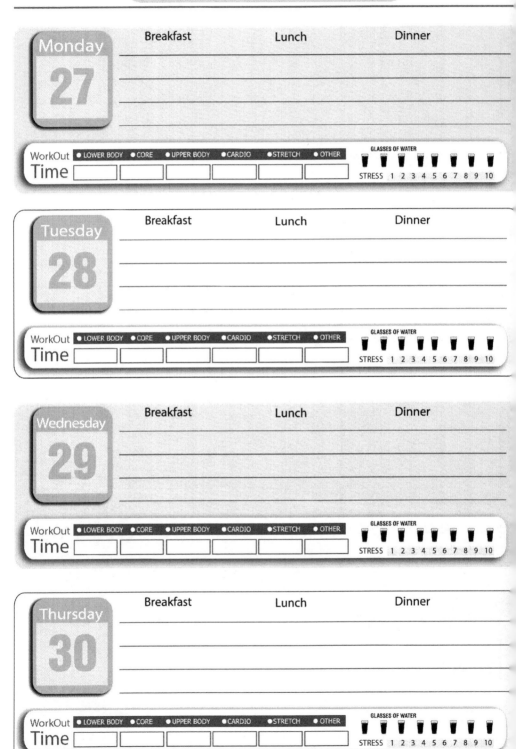

Monday 27

Breakfast   Lunch   Dinner

WorkOut   ● LOWER BODY   ● CORE   ● UPPER BODY   ● CARDIO   ● STRETCH   ● OTHER

Time

GLASSES OF WATER

STRESS   1   2   3   4   5   6   7   8   9   10

Tuesday 28

Breakfast   Lunch   Dinner

WorkOut   ● LOWER BODY   ● CORE   ● UPPER BODY   ● CARDIO   ● STRETCH   ● OTHER

Time

GLASSES OF WATER

STRESS   1   2   3   4   5   6   7   8   9   10

Wednesday 29

Breakfast   Lunch   Dinner

WorkOut   ● LOWER BODY   ● CORE   ● UPPER BODY   ● CARDIO   ● STRETCH   ● OTHER

Time

GLASSES OF WATER

STRESS   1   2   3   4   5   6   7   8   9   10

Thursday 30

Breakfast   Lunch   Dinner

WorkOut   ● LOWER BODY   ● CORE   ● UPPER BODY   ● CARDIO   ● STRETCH   ● OTHER

Time

GLASSES OF WATER

STRESS   1   2   3   4   5   6   7   8   9   10

Friday 1

Breakfast	Lunch	Dinner

WorkOut ● LOWER BODY ● CORE ● UPPER BODY ● CARDIO ● STRETCH ● OTHER

Time

GLASSES OF WATER

STRESS 1 2 3 4 5 6 7 8 9 10

Saturday 2

Breakfast	Lunch	Dinner

WorkOut ● LOWER BODY ● CORE ● UPPER BODY ● CARDIO ● STRETCH ● OTHER

Time

GLASSES OF WATER

STRESS 1 2 3 4 5 6 7 8 9 10

Sunday 3

Breakfast	Lunch	Dinner

WorkOut ● LOWER BODY ● CORE ● UPPER BODY ● CARDIO ● STRETCH ● OTHER

Time

GLASSES OF WATER

STRESS 1 2 3 4 5 6 7 8 9 10

This Month's Measurements:

Waist
Neck
Biceps
Chest
Hips
Thighs

Month Progress Report

Current Weight:

Notes:

July 2016

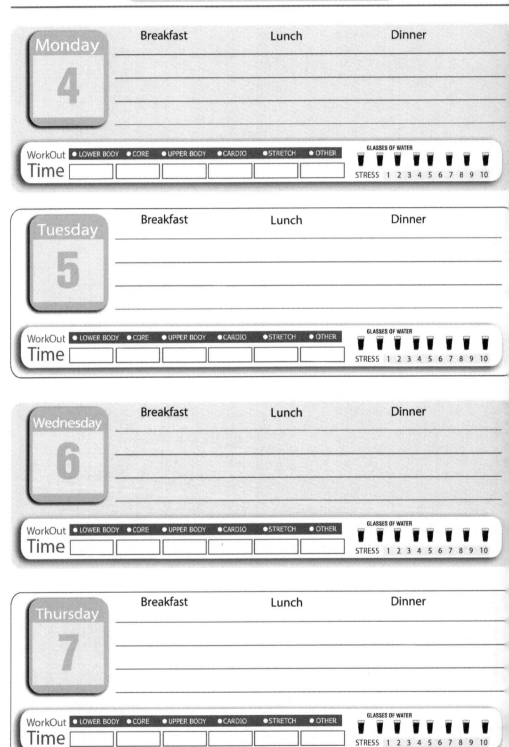

Monday 4

Breakfast	Lunch	Dinner

WorkOut ● LOWER BODY ● CORE ● UPPER BODY ● CARDIO ● STRETCH ● OTHER
Time

GLASSES OF WATER
STRESS 1 2 3 4 5 6 7 8 9 10

Tuesday 5

Breakfast	Lunch	Dinner

WorkOut ● LOWER BODY ● CORE ● UPPER BODY ● CARDIO ● STRETCH ● OTHER
Time

GLASSES OF WATER
STRESS 1 2 3 4 5 6 7 8 9 10

Wednesday 6

Breakfast	Lunch	Dinner

WorkOut ● LOWER BODY ● CORE ● UPPER BODY ● CARDIO ● STRETCH ● OTHER
Time

GLASSES OF WATER
STRESS 1 2 3 4 5 6 7 8 9 10

Thursday 7

Breakfast	Lunch	Dinner

WorkOut ● LOWER BODY ● CORE ● UPPER BODY ● CARDIO ● STRETCH ● OTHER
Time

GLASSES OF WATER
STRESS 1 2 3 4 5 6 7 8 9 10

Friday 8

Breakfast | Lunch | Dinner

WorkOut ● LOWER BODY ● CORE ● UPPER BODY ● CARDIO ● STRETCH ● OTHER
Time

GLASSES OF WATER
STRESS 1 2 3 4 5 6 7 8 9 10

Saturday 9

Breakfast | Lunch | Dinner

WorkOut ● LOWER BODY ● CORE ● UPPER BODY ● CARDIO ● STRETCH ● OTHER
Time

GLASSES OF WATER
STRESS 1 2 3 4 5 6 7 8 9 10

Sunday 10

Breakfast | Lunch | Dinner

WorkOut ● LOWER BODY ● CORE ● UPPER BODY ● CARDIO ● STRETCH ● OTHER
Time

GLASSES OF WATER
STRESS 1 2 3 4 5 6 7 8 9 10

Notes

Monday 11

Breakfast	Lunch	Dinner

WorkOut ● LOWER BODY ● CORE ● UPPER BODY ● CARDIO ● STRETCH ● OTHER

Time

GLASSES OF WATER

STRESS 1 2 3 4 5 6 7 8 9 10

Tuesday 12

Breakfast	Lunch	Dinner

WorkOut ● LOWER BODY ● CORE ● UPPER BODY ● CARDIO ● STRETCH ● OTHER

Time

GLASSES OF WATER

STRESS 1 2 3 4 5 6 7 8 9 10

Wednesday 13

Breakfast	Lunch	Dinner

WorkOut ● LOWER BODY ● CORE ● UPPER BODY ● CARDIO ● STRETCH ● OTHER

Time

GLASSES OF WATER

STRESS 1 2 3 4 5 6 7 8 9 10

Thursday 14

Breakfast	Lunch	Dinner

WorkOut ● LOWER BODY ● CORE ● UPPER BODY ● CARDIO ● STRETCH ● OTHER

Time

GLASSES OF WATER

STRESS 1 2 3 4 5 6 7 8 9 10

July 2016

Friday 15

Breakfast | Lunch | Dinner

WorkOut Time | ● LOWER BODY ● CORE ● UPPER BODY ● CARDIO ● STRETCH ● OTHER

GLASSES OF WATER
STRESS 1 2 3 4 5 6 7 8 9 10

Saturday 16

Breakfast | Lunch | Dinner

WorkOut Time | ● LOWER BODY ● CORE ● UPPER BODY ● CARDIO ● STRETCH ● OTHER

GLASSES OF WATER
STRESS 1 2 3 4 5 6 7 8 9 10

Sunday 17

Breakfast | Lunch | Dinner

WorkOut Time | ● LOWER BODY ● CORE ● UPPER BODY ● CARDIO ● STRETCH ● OTHER

GLASSES OF WATER
STRESS 1 2 3 4 5 6 7 8 9 10

Notes

Monday 18

Breakfast	Lunch	Dinner

WorkOut ● LOWER BODY ● CORE ● UPPER BODY ● CARDIO ● STRETCH ● OTHER

Time

GLASSES OF WATER

STRESS 1 2 3 4 5 6 7 8 9 10

Tuesday 19

Breakfast	Lunch	Dinner

WorkOut ● LOWER BODY ● CORE ● UPPER BODY ● CARDIO ● STRETCH ● OTHER

Time

GLASSES OF WATER

STRESS 1 2 3 4 5 6 7 8 9 10

Wednesday 20

Breakfast	Lunch	Dinner

WorkOut ● LOWER BODY ● CORE ● UPPER BODY ● CARDIO ● STRETCH ● OTHER

Time

GLASSES OF WATER

STRESS 1 2 3 4 5 6 7 8 9 10

Thursday 21

Breakfast	Lunch	Dinner

WorkOut ● LOWER BODY ● CORE ● UPPER BODY ● CARDIO ● STRETCH ● OTHER

Time

GLASSES OF WATER

STRESS 1 2 3 4 5 6 7 8 9 10

Friday 22

Breakfast	Lunch	Dinner

WorkOut Time · LOWER BODY · CORE · UPPER BODY · CARDIO · STRETCH · OTHER

GLASSES OF WATER

STRESS 1 2 3 4 5 6 7 8 9 10

Saturday 23

Breakfast	Lunch	Dinner

WorkOut Time · LOWER BODY · CORE · UPPER BODY · CARDIO · STRETCH · OTHER

GLASSES OF WATER

STRESS 1 2 3 4 5 6 7 8 9 10

Sunday 24

Breakfast	Lunch	Dinner

WorkOut Time · LOWER BODY · CORE · UPPER BODY · CARDIO · STRETCH · OTHER

GLASSES OF WATER

STRESS 1 2 3 4 5 6 7 8 9 10

Notes

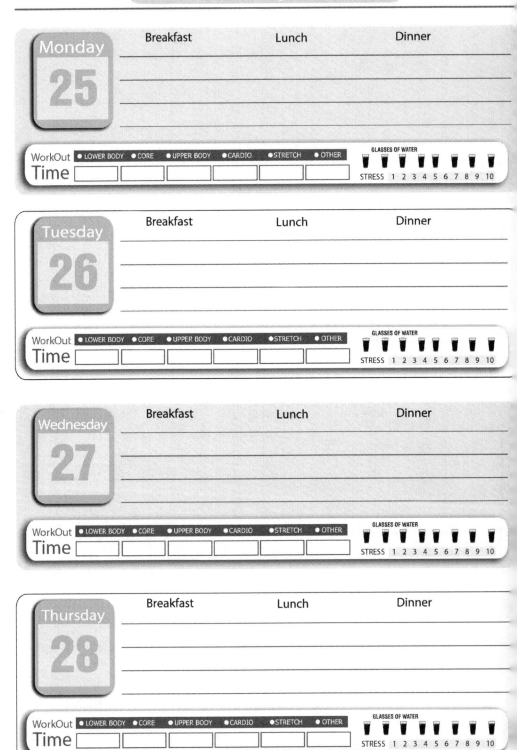

July
2016

Monday
25

Breakfast   Lunch   Dinner

WorkOut   ● LOWER BODY   ● CORE   ● UPPER BODY   ● CARDIO   ● STRETCH   ● OTHER
Time

GLASSES OF WATER
STRESS   1 2 3 4 5 6 7 8 9 10

Tuesday
26

Breakfast   Lunch   Dinner

WorkOut   ● LOWER BODY   ● CORE   ● UPPER BODY   ● CARDIO   ● STRETCH   ● OTHER
Time

GLASSES OF WATER
STRESS   1 2 3 4 5 6 7 8 9 10

Wednesday
27

Breakfast   Lunch   Dinner

WorkOut   ● LOWER BODY   ● CORE   ● UPPER BODY   ● CARDIO   ● STRETCH   ● OTHER
Time

GLASSES OF WATER
STRESS   1 2 3 4 5 6 7 8 9 10

Thursday
28

Breakfast   Lunch   Dinner

WorkOut   ● LOWER BODY   ● CORE   ● UPPER BODY   ● CARDIO   ● STRETCH   ● OTHER
Time

GLASSES OF WATER
STRESS   1 2 3 4 5 6 7 8 9 10

Friday 29

	Breakfast	Lunch	Dinner

WorkOut ● LOWER BODY ● CORE ● UPPER BODY ● CARDIO ● STRETCH ● OTHER

Time

GLASSES OF WATER

STRESS 1 2 3 4 5 6 7 8 9 10

Saturday 30

	Breakfast	Lunch	Dinner

WorkOut ● LOWER BODY ● CORE ● UPPER BODY ● CARDIO ● STRETCH ● OTHER

Time

GLASSES OF WATER

STRESS 1 2 3 4 5 6 7 8 9 10

Sunday 31

	Breakfast	Lunch	Dinner

WorkOut ● LOWER BODY ● CORE ● UPPER BODY ● CARDIO ● STRETCH ● OTHER

Time

GLASSES OF WATER

STRESS 1 2 3 4 5 6 7 8 9 10

This Month's Measurements:

Waist
Neck
Biceps
Chest
Hips
Thighs

Month Progress Report

Current Weight:

Notes:

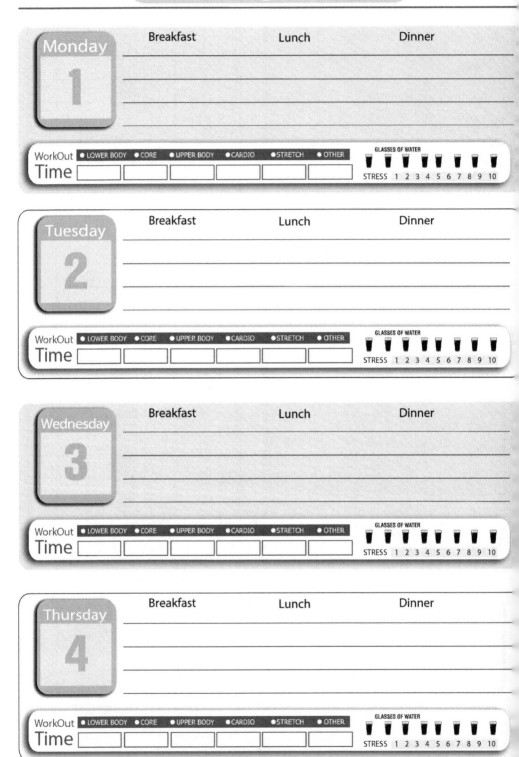

August 2016

Monday 1

Breakfast | Lunch | Dinner

WorkOut — ● LOWER BODY ● CORE ● UPPER BODY ● CARDIO ● STRETCH ● OTHER
Time

GLASSES OF WATER
STRESS 1 2 3 4 5 6 7 8 9 10

Tuesday 2

Breakfast | Lunch | Dinner

WorkOut — ● LOWER BODY ● CORE ● UPPER BODY ● CARDIO ● STRETCH ● OTHER
Time

GLASSES OF WATER
STRESS 1 2 3 4 5 6 7 8 9 10

Wednesday 3

Breakfast | Lunch | Dinner

WorkOut — ● LOWER BODY ● CORE ● UPPER BODY ● CARDIO ● STRETCH ● OTHER
Time

GLASSES OF WATER
STRESS 1 2 3 4 5 6 7 8 9 10

Thursday 4

Breakfast | Lunch | Dinner

WorkOut — ● LOWER BODY ● CORE ● UPPER BODY ● CARDIO ● STRETCH ● OTHER
Time

GLASSES OF WATER
STRESS 1 2 3 4 5 6 7 8 9 10

Friday 5

Breakfast	Lunch	Dinner

WorkOut Time
● LOWER BODY ● CORE ● UPPER BODY ● CARDIO ● STRETCH ● OTHER

GLASSES OF WATER
STRESS 1 2 3 4 5 6 7 8 9 10

Saturday 6

Breakfast	Lunch	Dinner

WorkOut Time
● LOWER BODY ● CORE ● UPPER BODY ● CARDIO ● STRETCH ● OTHER

GLASSES OF WATER
STRESS 1 2 3 4 5 6 7 8 9 10

Sunday 7

Breakfast	Lunch	Dinner

WorkOut Time
● LOWER BODY ● CORE ● UPPER BODY ● CARDIO ● STRETCH ● OTHER

GLASSES OF WATER
STRESS 1 2 3 4 5 6 7 8 9 10

Notes

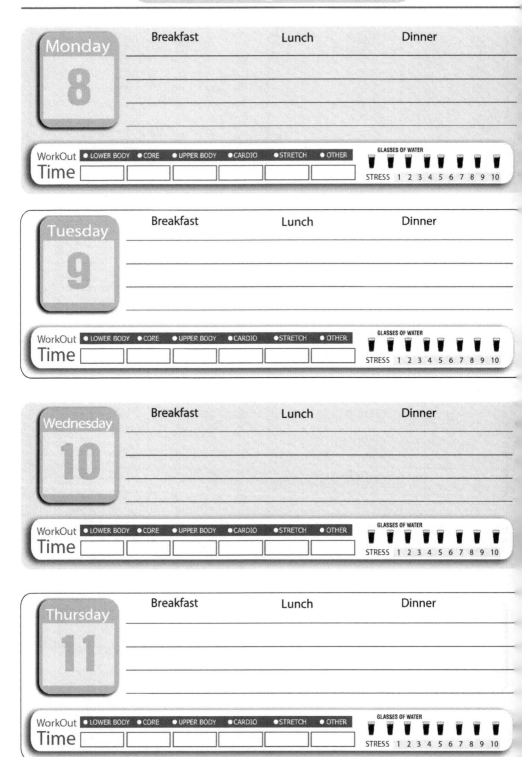

Monday 8

Breakfast	Lunch	Dinner

WorkOut Time — ● LOWER BODY ● CORE ● UPPER BODY ● CARDIO ● STRETCH ● OTHER

GLASSES OF WATER

STRESS 1 2 3 4 5 6 7 8 9 10

Tuesday 9

Breakfast	Lunch	Dinner

WorkOut Time — ● LOWER BODY ● CORE ● UPPER BODY ● CARDIO ● STRETCH ● OTHER

GLASSES OF WATER

STRESS 1 2 3 4 5 6 7 8 9 10

Wednesday 10

Breakfast	Lunch	Dinner

WorkOut Time — ● LOWER BODY ● CORE ● UPPER BODY ● CARDIO ● STRETCH ● OTHER

GLASSES OF WATER

STRESS 1 2 3 4 5 6 7 8 9 10

Thursday 11

Breakfast	Lunch	Dinner

WorkOut Time — ● LOWER BODY ● CORE ● UPPER BODY ● CARDIO ● STRETCH ● OTHER

GLASSES OF WATER

STRESS 1 2 3 4 5 6 7 8 9 10

August 2016

Friday 12

Breakfast
Lunch
Dinner
_____
_____
_____
_____

WorkOut Time | ●LOWER BODY ●CORE ●UPPER BODY ●CARDIO ●STRETCH ●OTHER
GLASSES OF WATER
STRESS 1 2 3 4 5 6 7 8 9 10

Saturday 13

Breakfast
Lunch
Dinner
_____
_____
_____
_____

WorkOut Time | ●LOWER BODY ●CORE ●UPPER BODY ●CARDIO ●STRETCH ●OTHER
GLASSES OF WATER
STRESS 1 2 3 4 5 6 7 8 9 10

Sunday 14

Breakfast
Lunch
Dinner
_____
_____
_____
_____

WorkOut Time | ●LOWER BODY ●CORE ●UPPER BODY ●CARDIO ●STRETCH ●OTHER
GLASSES OF WATER
STRESS 1 2 3 4 5 6 7 8 9 10

Notes

Monday 15

Breakfast | Lunch | Dinner

WorkOut ●LOWER BODY ●CORE ●UPPER BODY ●CARDIO ●STRETCH ●OTHER
Time

GLASSES OF WATER
STRESS 1 2 3 4 5 6 7 8 9 10

Tuesday 16

Breakfast | Lunch | Dinner

WorkOut ●LOWER BODY ●CORE ●UPPER BODY ●CARDIO ●STRETCH ●OTHER
Time

GLASSES OF WATER
STRESS 1 2 3 4 5 6 7 8 9 10

Wednesday 17

Breakfast | Lunch | Dinner

WorkOut ●LOWER BODY ●CORE ●UPPER BODY ●CARDIO ●STRETCH ●OTHER
Time

GLASSES OF WATER
STRESS 1 2 3 4 5 6 7 8 9 10

Thursday 18

Breakfast | Lunch | Dinner

WorkOut ●LOWER BODY ●CORE ●UPPER BODY ●CARDIO ●STRETCH ●OTHER
Time

GLASSES OF WATER
STRESS 1 2 3 4 5 6 7 8 9 10

Friday 19

Breakfast	Lunch	Dinner

WorkOut Time

● LOWER BODY ● CORE ● UPPER BODY ● CARDIO ● STRETCH ● OTHER

GLASSES OF WATER

STRESS 1 2 3 4 5 6 7 8 9 10

Saturday 20

Breakfast	Lunch	Dinner

WorkOut Time

● LOWER BODY ● CORE ● UPPER BODY ● CARDIO ● STRETCH ● OTHER

GLASSES OF WATER

STRESS 1 2 3 4 5 6 7 8 9 10

Sunday 21

Breakfast	Lunch	Dinner

WorkOut Time

● LOWER BODY ● CORE ● UPPER BODY ● CARDIO ● STRETCH ● OTHER

GLASSES OF WATER

STRESS 1 2 3 4 5 6 7 8 9 10

Notes

Monday 22

Breakfast   Lunch   Dinner

_____
_____
_____
_____

WorkOut ● LOWER BODY ● CORE ● UPPER BODY ● CARDIO ● STRETCH ● OTHER

Time [   ] [   ] [   ] [   ] [   ] [   ]

GLASSES OF WATER
STRESS 1 2 3 4 5 6 7 8 9 10

Tuesday 23

Breakfast   Lunch   Dinner

_____
_____
_____
_____

WorkOut ● LOWER BODY ● CORE ● UPPER BODY ● CARDIO ● STRETCH ● OTHER

Time [   ] [   ] [   ] [   ] [   ] [   ]

GLASSES OF WATER
STRESS 1 2 3 4 5 6 7 8 9 10

Wednesday 24

Breakfast   Lunch   Dinner

_____
_____
_____
_____

WorkOut ● LOWER BODY ● CORE ● UPPER BODY ● CARDIO ● STRETCH ● OTHER

Time [   ] [   ] [   ] [   ] [   ] [   ]

GLASSES OF WATER
STRESS 1 2 3 4 5 6 7 8 9 10

Thursday 25

Breakfast   Lunch   Dinner

_____
_____
_____
_____

WorkOut ● LOWER BODY ● CORE ● UPPER BODY ● CARDIO ● STRETCH ● OTHER

Time [   ] [   ] [   ] [   ] [   ] [   ]

GLASSES OF WATER
STRESS 1 2 3 4 5 6 7 8 9 10

Friday 26

Breakfast   Lunch   Dinner

_____
_____
_____
_____

WorkOut ● LOWER BODY ● CORE ● UPPER BODY ● CARDIO ● STRETCH ● OTHER

Time [____] [____] [____] [____] [____] [____]

GLASSES OF WATER

STRESS 1 2 3 4 5 6 7 8 9 10

Saturday 27

Breakfast   Lunch   Dinner

_____
_____
_____
_____

WorkOut ● LOWER BODY ● CORE ● UPPER BODY ● CARDIO ● STRETCH ● OTHER

Time [____] [____] [____] [____] [____] [____]

GLASSES OF WATER

STRESS 1 2 3 4 5 6 7 8 9 10

Sunday 28

Breakfast   Lunch   Dinner

_____
_____
_____
_____

WorkOut ● LOWER BODY ● CORE ● UPPER BODY ● CARDIO ● STRETCH ● OTHER

Time [____] [____] [____] [____] [____] [____]

GLASSES OF WATER

STRESS 1 2 3 4 5 6 7 8 9 10

Notes

_____
_____
_____
_____

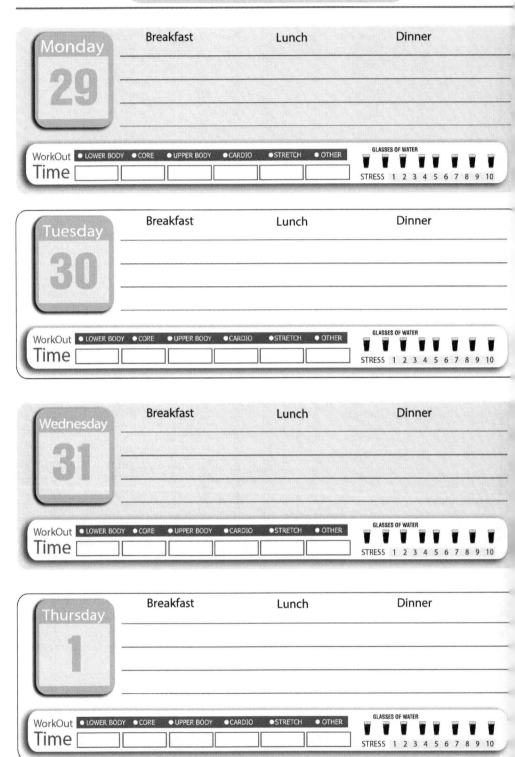

Monday 29

Breakfast   Lunch   Dinner

WorkOut
Time
● LOWER BODY ● CORE ● UPPER BODY ● CARDIO ● STRETCH ● OTHER

GLASSES OF WATER
STRESS 1 2 3 4 5 6 7 8 9 10

Tuesday 30

Breakfast   Lunch   Dinner

WorkOut
Time
● LOWER BODY ● CORE ● UPPER BODY ● CARDIO ● STRETCH ● OTHER

GLASSES OF WATER
STRESS 1 2 3 4 5 6 7 8 9 10

Wednesday 31

Breakfast   Lunch   Dinner

WorkOut
Time
● LOWER BODY ● CORE ● UPPER BODY ● CARDIO ● STRETCH ● OTHER

GLASSES OF WATER
STRESS 1 2 3 4 5 6 7 8 9 10

Thursday 1

Breakfast   Lunch   Dinner

WorkOut
Time
● LOWER BODY ● CORE ● UPPER BODY ● CARDIO ● STRETCH ● OTHER

GLASSES OF WATER
STRESS 1 2 3 4 5 6 7 8 9 10

Friday 2

	Breakfast	Lunch	Dinner

WorkOut ● LOWER BODY ● CORE ● UPPER BODY ● CARDIO ● STRETCH ● OTHER

Time

GLASSES OF WATER
STRESS 1 2 3 4 5 6 7 8 9 10

Saturday 3

	Breakfast	Lunch	Dinner

WorkOut ● LOWER BODY ● CORE ● UPPER BODY ● CARDIO ● STRETCH ● OTHER

Time

GLASSES OF WATER
STRESS 1 2 3 4 5 6 7 8 9 10

Sunday 4

	Breakfast	Lunch	Dinner

WorkOut ● LOWER BODY ● CORE ● UPPER BODY ● CARDIO ● STRETCH ● OTHER

Time

GLASSES OF WATER
STRESS 1 2 3 4 5 6 7 8 9 10

This Month's Measurements:

Waist
Neck
Biceps
Chest
Hips
Thighs

Month Progress Report

Current Weight:

Notes:

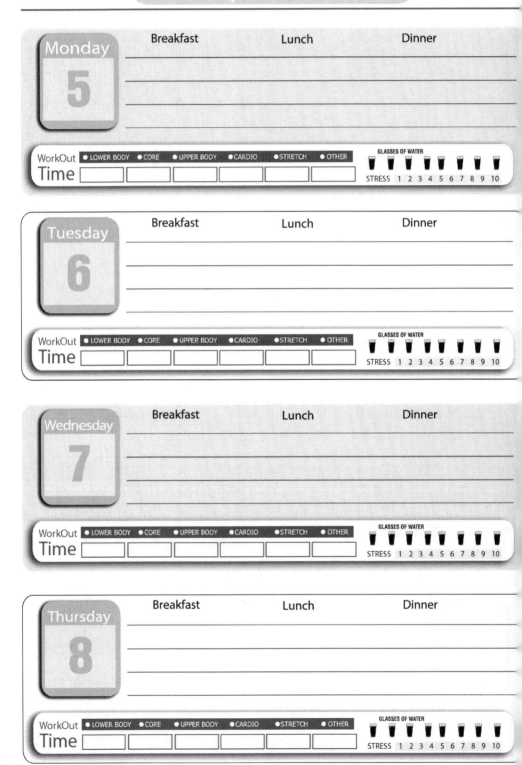

Monday 5

Breakfast Lunch Dinner

WorkOut Time ● LOWER BODY ● CORE ● UPPER BODY ● CARDIO ● STRETCH ● OTHER

GLASSES OF WATER

STRESS 1 2 3 4 5 6 7 8 9 10

Tuesday 6

Breakfast Lunch Dinner

WorkOut Time ● LOWER BODY ● CORE ● UPPER BODY ● CARDIO ● STRETCH ● OTHER

GLASSES OF WATER

STRESS 1 2 3 4 5 6 7 8 9 10

Wednesday 7

Breakfast Lunch Dinner

WorkOut Time ● LOWER BODY ● CORE ● UPPER BODY ● CARDIO ● STRETCH ● OTHER

GLASSES OF WATER

STRESS 1 2 3 4 5 6 7 8 9 10

Thursday 8

Breakfast Lunch Dinner

WorkOut Time ● LOWER BODY ● CORE ● UPPER BODY ● CARDIO ● STRETCH ● OTHER

GLASSES OF WATER

STRESS 1 2 3 4 5 6 7 8 9 10

September 2016

Friday 9

Breakfast | Lunch | Dinner

WorkOut Time | ● LOWER BODY ● CORE ● UPPER BODY ● CARDIO ● STRETCH ● OTHER

GLASSES OF WATER
STRESS 1 2 3 4 5 6 7 8 9 10

Saturday 10

Breakfast | Lunch | Dinner

WorkOut Time | ● LOWER BODY ● CORE ● UPPER BODY ● CARDIO ● STRETCH ● OTHER

GLASSES OF WATER
STRESS 1 2 3 4 5 6 7 8 9 10

Sunday 11

Breakfast | Lunch | Dinner

WorkOut Time | ● LOWER BODY ● CORE ● UPPER BODY ● CARDIO ● STRETCH ● OTHER

GLASSES OF WATER
STRESS 1 2 3 4 5 6 7 8 9 10

Notes

September 2016

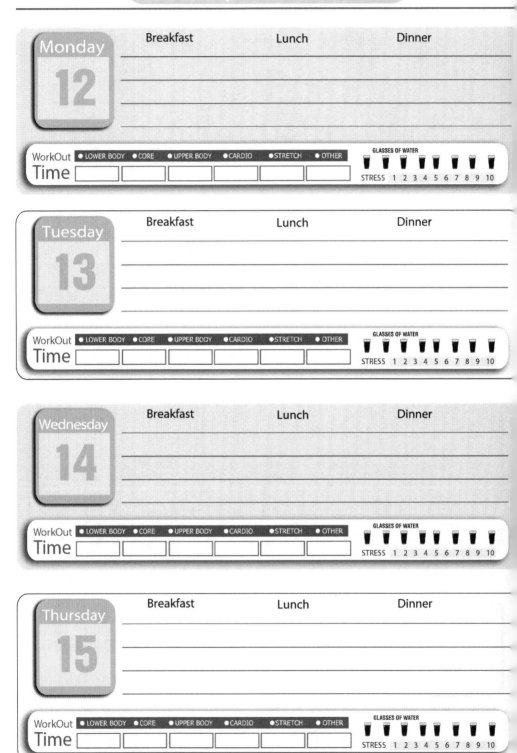

Monday 12

Breakfast	Lunch	Dinner

WorkOut ● LOWER BODY ● CORE ● UPPER BODY ● CARDIO ● STRETCH ● OTHER
Time

GLASSES OF WATER
STRESS 1 2 3 4 5 6 7 8 9 10

Tuesday 13

Breakfast	Lunch	Dinner

WorkOut ● LOWER BODY ● CORE ● UPPER BODY ● CARDIO ● STRETCH ● OTHER
Time

GLASSES OF WATER
STRESS 1 2 3 4 5 6 7 8 9 10

Wednesday 14

Breakfast	Lunch	Dinner

WorkOut ● LOWER BODY ● CORE ● UPPER BODY ● CARDIO ● STRETCH ● OTHER
Time

GLASSES OF WATER
STRESS 1 2 3 4 5 6 7 8 9 10

Thursday 15

Breakfast	Lunch	Dinner

WorkOut ● LOWER BODY ● CORE ● UPPER BODY ● CARDIO ● STRETCH ● OTHER
Time

GLASSES OF WATER
STRESS 1 2 3 4 5 6 7 8 9 10

Friday 16

Breakfast	Lunch	Dinner

WorkOut Time: ● LOWER BODY ● CORE ● UPPER BODY ● CARDIO ● STRETCH ● OTHER

GLASSES OF WATER
STRESS 1 2 3 4 5 6 7 8 9 10

Saturday 17

Breakfast	Lunch	Dinner

WorkOut Time: ● LOWER BODY ● CORE ● UPPER BODY ● CARDIO ● STRETCH ● OTHER

GLASSES OF WATER
STRESS 1 2 3 4 5 6 7 8 9 10

Sunday 18

Breakfast	Lunch	Dinner

WorkOut Time: ● LOWER BODY ● CORE ● UPPER BODY ● CARDIO ● STRETCH ● OTHER

GLASSES OF WATER
STRESS 1 2 3 4 5 6 7 8 9 10

Notes

September 2016

Monday 19

Breakfast   Lunch   Dinner

WorkOut ● LOWER BODY ● CORE ● UPPER BODY ● CARDIO ● STRETCH ● OTHER
Time
GLASSES OF WATER
STRESS 1 2 3 4 5 6 7 8 9 10

Tuesday 20

Breakfast   Lunch   Dinner

WorkOut ● LOWER BODY ● CORE ● UPPER BODY ● CARDIO ● STRETCH ● OTHER
Time
GLASSES OF WATER
STRESS 1 2 3 4 5 6 7 8 9 10

Wednesday 21

Breakfast   Lunch   Dinner

WorkOut ● LOWER BODY ● CORE ● UPPER BODY ● CARDIO ● STRETCH ● OTHER
Time
GLASSES OF WATER
STRESS 1 2 3 4 5 6 7 8 9 10

Thursday 22

Breakfast   Lunch   Dinner

WorkOut ● LOWER BODY ● CORE ● UPPER BODY ● CARDIO ● STRETCH ● OTHER
Time
GLASSES OF WATER
STRESS 1 2 3 4 5 6 7 8 9 10

Friday
23

Breakfast   **Lunch**   **Dinner**

WorkOut ● LOWER BODY ● CORE ● UPPER BODY ● CARDIO ● STRETCH ● OTHER

GLASSES OF WATER

Time

STRESS 1 2 3 4 5 6 7 8 9 10

Saturday
24

Breakfast   **Lunch**   **Dinner**

WorkOut ● LOWER BODY ● CORE ● UPPER BODY ● CARDIO ● STRETCH ● OTHER

GLASSES OF WATER

Time

STRESS 1 2 3 4 5 6 7 8 9 10

Sunday
25

Breakfast   **Lunch**   **Dinner**

WorkOut ● LOWER BODY ● CORE ● UPPER BODY ● CARDIO ● STRETCH ● OTHER

GLASSES OF WATER

Time

STRESS 1 2 3 4 5 6 7 8 9 10

Notes

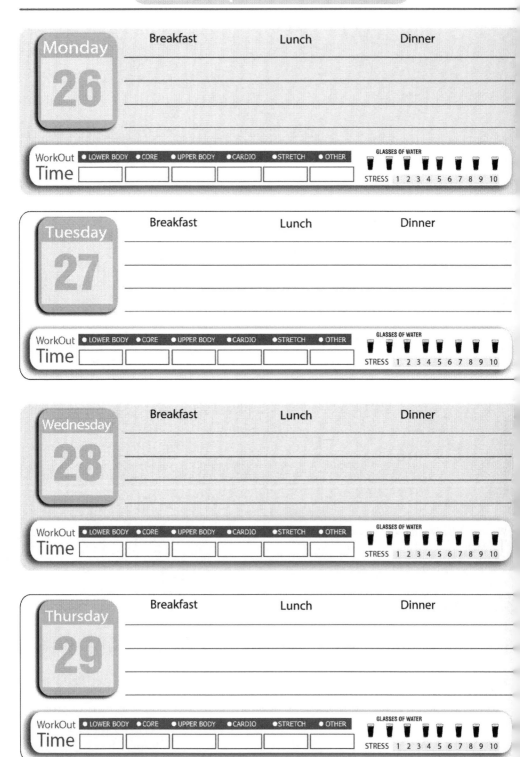

Monday 26

Breakfast Lunch Dinner

WorkOut | LOWER BODY | CORE | UPPER BODY | CARDIO | STRETCH | OTHER
Time

GLASSES OF WATER
STRESS 1 2 3 4 5 6 7 8 9 10

Tuesday 27

Breakfast Lunch Dinner

WorkOut | LOWER BODY | CORE | UPPER BODY | CARDIO | STRETCH | OTHER
Time

GLASSES OF WATER
STRESS 1 2 3 4 5 6 7 8 9 10

Wednesday 28

Breakfast Lunch Dinner

WorkOut | LOWER BODY | CORE | UPPER BODY | CARDIO | STRETCH | OTHER
Time

GLASSES OF WATER
STRESS 1 2 3 4 5 6 7 8 9 10

Thursday 29

Breakfast Lunch Dinner

WorkOut | LOWER BODY | CORE | UPPER BODY | CARDIO | STRETCH | OTHER
Time

GLASSES OF WATER
STRESS 1 2 3 4 5 6 7 8 9 10

Friday 30

	Breakfast	Lunch	Dinner

WorkOut ● LOWER BODY ● CORE ● UPPER BODY ● CARDIO ● STRETCH ● OTHER

Time

GLASSES OF WATER

STRESS 1 2 3 4 5 6 7 8 9 10

Saturday 1

	Breakfast	Lunch	Dinner

WorkOut ● LOWER BODY ● CORE ● UPPER BODY ● CARDIO ● STRETCH ● OTHER

Time

GLASSES OF WATER

STRESS 1 2 3 4 5 6 7 8 9 10

Sunday 2

	Breakfast	Lunch	Dinner

WorkOut ● LOWER BODY ● CORE ● UPPER BODY ● CARDIO ● STRETCH ● OTHER

Time

GLASSES OF WATER

STRESS 1 2 3 4 5 6 7 8 9 10

This Month's Measurements:

Waist
Neck
Biceps
Chest
Hips
Thighs

Month Progress Report

Current Weight:

Notes:

Monday 3

Breakfast	Lunch	Dinner

WorkOut ● LOWER BODY ● CORE ● UPPER BODY ● CARDIO ● STRETCH ● OTHER

Time

GLASSES OF WATER

STRESS 1 2 3 4 5 6 7 8 9 10

Tuesday 4

Breakfast	Lunch	Dinner

WorkOut ● LOWER BODY ● CORE ● UPPER BODY ● CARDIO ● STRETCH ● OTHER

Time

GLASSES OF WATER

STRESS 1 2 3 4 5 6 7 8 9 10

Wednesday 5

Breakfast	Lunch	Dinner

WorkOut ● LOWER BODY ● CORE ● UPPER BODY ● CARDIO ● STRETCH ● OTHER

Time

GLASSES OF WATER

STRESS 1 2 3 4 5 6 7 8 9 10

Thursday 6

Breakfast	Lunch	Dinner

WorkOut ● LOWER BODY ● CORE ● UPPER BODY ● CARDIO ● STRETCH ● OTHER

Time

GLASSES OF WATER

STRESS 1 2 3 4 5 6 7 8 9 10

Friday 7

Breakfast	Lunch	Dinner

WorkOut ● LOWER BODY ● CORE ● UPPER BODY ● CARDIO ● STRETCH ● OTHER

Time ☐ ☐ ☐ ☐ ☐ ☐

GLASSES OF WATER

STRESS 1 2 3 4 5 6 7 8 9 10

Saturday 8

Breakfast	Lunch	Dinner

WorkOut ● LOWER BODY ● CORE ● UPPER BODY ● CARDIO ● STRETCH ● OTHER

Time ☐ ☐ ☐ ☐ ☐ ☐

GLASSES OF WATER

STRESS 1 2 3 4 5 6 7 8 9 10

Sunday 9

Breakfast	Lunch	Dinner

WorkOut ● LOWER BODY ● CORE ● UPPER BODY ● CARDIO ● STRETCH ● OTHER

Time ☐ ☐ ☐ ☐ ☐ ☐

GLASSES OF WATER

STRESS 1 2 3 4 5 6 7 8 9 10

Notes

Monday 10

	Breakfast	Lunch	Dinner

WorkOut ● LOWER BODY ● CORE ● UPPER BODY ● CARDIO ● STRETCH ● OTHER

Time

GLASSES OF WATER

STRESS 1 2 3 4 5 6 7 8 9 10

Tuesday 11

	Breakfast	Lunch	Dinner

WorkOut ● LOWER BODY ● CORE ● UPPER BODY ● CARDIO ● STRETCH ● OTHER

Time

GLASSES OF WATER

STRESS 1 2 3 4 5 6 7 8 9 10

Wednesday 12

	Breakfast	Lunch	Dinner

WorkOut ● LOWER BODY ● CORE ● UPPER BODY ● CARDIO ● STRETCH ● OTHER

Time

GLASSES OF WATER

STRESS 1 2 3 4 5 6 7 8 9 10

Thursday 13

	Breakfast	Lunch	Dinner

WorkOut ● LOWER BODY ● CORE ● UPPER BODY ● CARDIO ● STRETCH ● OTHER

Time

GLASSES OF WATER

STRESS 1 2 3 4 5 6 7 8 9 10

Friday 14

Breakfast	Lunch	Dinner

WorkOut Time ● LOWER BODY ● CORE ● UPPER BODY ● CARDIO ● STRETCH ● OTHER

GLASSES OF WATER
STRESS 1 2 3 4 5 6 7 8 9 10

Saturday 15

Breakfast	Lunch	Dinner

WorkOut Time ● LOWER BODY ● CORE ● UPPER BODY ● CARDIO ● STRETCH ● OTHER

GLASSES OF WATER
STRESS 1 2 3 4 5 6 7 8 9 10

Sunday 16

Breakfast	Lunch	Dinner

WorkOut Time ● LOWER BODY ● CORE ● UPPER BODY ● CARDIO ● STRETCH ● OTHER

GLASSES OF WATER
STRESS 1 2 3 4 5 6 7 8 9 10

Notes

Monday 17

Breakfast	Lunch	Dinner

WorkOut ● LOWER BODY ● CORE ● UPPER BODY ● CARDIO ● STRETCH ● OTHER

Time [ ] [ ] [ ] [ ] [ ] [ ]

GLASSES OF WATER

STRESS 1 2 3 4 5 6 7 8 9 10

Tuesday 18

Breakfast	Lunch	Dinner

WorkOut ● LOWER BODY ● CORE ● UPPER BODY ● CARDIO ● STRETCH ● OTHER

Time [ ] [ ] [ ] [ ] [ ] [ ]

GLASSES OF WATER

STRESS 1 2 3 4 5 6 7 8 9 10

Wednesday 19

Breakfast	Lunch	Dinner

WorkOut ● LOWER BODY ● CORE ● UPPER BODY ● CARDIO ● STRETCH ● OTHER

Time [ ] [ ] [ ] [ ] [ ] [ ]

GLASSES OF WATER

STRESS 1 2 3 4 5 6 7 8 9 10

Thursday 20

Breakfast	Lunch	Dinner

WorkOut ● LOWER BODY ● CORE ● UPPER BODY ● CARDIO ● STRETCH ● OTHER

Time [ ] [ ] [ ] [ ] [ ] [ ]

GLASSES OF WATER

STRESS 1 2 3 4 5 6 7 8 9 10

Friday 21

Breakfast	Lunch	Dinner

WorkOut Time — ● LOWER BODY ● CORE ● UPPER BODY ● CARDIO ● STRETCH ● OTHER

GLASSES OF WATER

STRESS 1 2 3 4 5 6 7 8 9 10

Saturday 22

Breakfast	Lunch	Dinner

WorkOut Time — ● LOWER BODY ● CORE ● UPPER BODY ● CARDIO ● STRETCH ● OTHER

GLASSES OF WATER

STRESS 1 2 3 4 5 6 7 8 9 10

Sunday 23

Breakfast	Lunch	Dinner

WorkOut Time — ● LOWER BODY ● CORE ● UPPER BODY ● CARDIO ● STRETCH ● OTHER

GLASSES OF WATER

STRESS 1 2 3 4 5 6 7 8 9 10

Notes

Monday 24

	Breakfast	Lunch	Dinner

WorkOut ● LOWER BODY ● CORE ● UPPER BODY ● CARDIO ● STRETCH ● OTHER

Time

GLASSES OF WATER

STRESS 1 2 3 4 5 6 7 8 9 10

Tuesday 25

	Breakfast	Lunch	Dinner

WorkOut ● LOWER BODY ● CORE ● UPPER BODY ● CARDIO ● STRETCH ● OTHER

Time

GLASSES OF WATER

STRESS 1 2 3 4 5 6 7 8 9 10

Wednesday 26

	Breakfast	Lunch	Dinner

WorkOut ● LOWER BODY ● CORE ● UPPER BODY ● CARDIO ● STRETCH ● OTHER

Time

GLASSES OF WATER

STRESS 1 2 3 4 5 6 7 8 9 10

Thursday 27

	Breakfast	Lunch	Dinner

WorkOut ● LOWER BODY ● CORE ● UPPER BODY ● CARDIO ● STRETCH ● OTHER

Time

GLASSES OF WATER

STRESS 1 2 3 4 5 6 7 8 9 10

October 2016

Friday 28
Breakfast ___ Lunch ___ Dinner ___

WorkOut ● LOWER BODY ● CORE ● UPPER BODY ● CARDIO ● STRETCH ● OTHER
Time [ ] [ ] [ ] [ ] [ ] [ ]
GLASSES OF WATER
STRESS 1 2 3 4 5 6 7 8 9 10

Saturday 29
Breakfast ___ Lunch ___ Dinner ___

WorkOut ● LOWER BODY ● CORE ● UPPER BODY ● CARDIO ● STRETCH ● OTHER
Time [ ] [ ] [ ] [ ] [ ] [ ]
GLASSES OF WATER
STRESS 1 2 3 4 5 6 7 8 9 10

Sunday 30
Breakfast ___ Lunch ___ Dinner ___

WorkOut ● LOWER BODY ● CORE ● UPPER BODY ● CARDIO ● STRETCH ● OTHER
Time [ ] [ ] [ ] [ ] [ ] [ ]
GLASSES OF WATER
STRESS 1 2 3 4 5 6 7 8 9 10

This Month's Measurements:
Waist [ ]
Neck [ ]
Biceps [ ]
Chest [ ]
Hips [ ]
Thighs [ ]

Month Progress Report
Current Weight: [ ]
Notes: ___

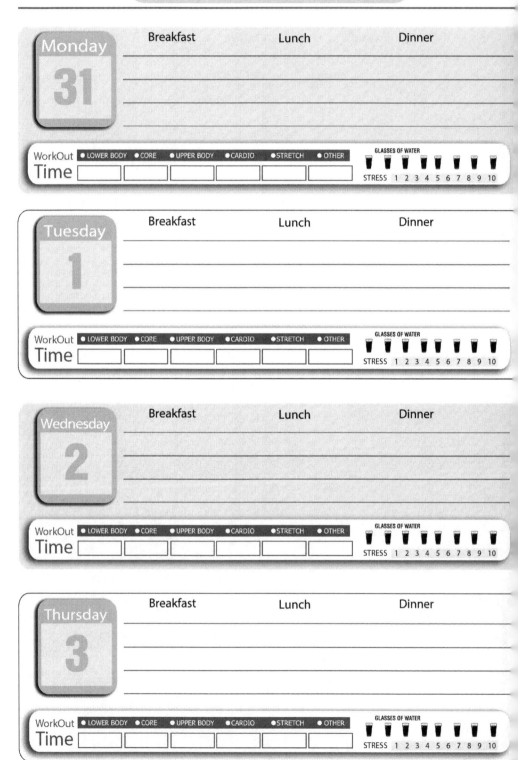

Monday 31

Breakfast   Lunch   Dinner

WorkOut Time — LOWER BODY ● CORE ● UPPER BODY ● CARDIO ● STRETCH ● OTHER

GLASSES OF WATER

STRESS 1 2 3 4 5 6 7 8 9 10

Tuesday 1

Breakfast   Lunch   Dinner

WorkOut Time — LOWER BODY ● CORE ● UPPER BODY ● CARDIO ● STRETCH ● OTHER

GLASSES OF WATER

STRESS 1 2 3 4 5 6 7 8 9 10

Wednesday 2

Breakfast   Lunch   Dinner

WorkOut Time — LOWER BODY ● CORE ● UPPER BODY ● CARDIO ● STRETCH ● OTHER

GLASSES OF WATER

STRESS 1 2 3 4 5 6 7 8 9 10

Thursday 3

Breakfast   Lunch   Dinner

WorkOut Time — LOWER BODY ● CORE ● UPPER BODY ● CARDIO ● STRETCH ● OTHER

GLASSES OF WATER

STRESS 1 2 3 4 5 6 7 8 9 10

Friday 4

Breakfast	Lunch	Dinner
_____	_____	_____
_____	_____	_____
_____	_____	_____
_____	_____	_____

WorkOut ● LOWER BODY ● CORE ● UPPER BODY ● CARDIO ● STRETCH ● OTHER
Time [ ] [ ] [ ] [ ] [ ] [ ]

GLASSES OF WATER
STRESS 1 2 3 4 5 6 7 8 9 10

Saturday 5

Breakfast	Lunch	Dinner
_____	_____	_____
_____	_____	_____
_____	_____	_____
_____	_____	_____

WorkOut ● LOWER BODY ● CORE ● UPPER BODY ● CARDIO ● STRETCH ● OTHER
Time [ ] [ ] [ ] [ ] [ ] [ ]

GLASSES OF WATER
STRESS 1 2 3 4 5 6 7 8 9 10

Sunday 6

Breakfast	Lunch	Dinner
_____	_____	_____
_____	_____	_____
_____	_____	_____
_____	_____	_____

WorkOut ● LOWER BODY ● CORE ● UPPER BODY ● CARDIO ● STRETCH ● OTHER
Time [ ] [ ] [ ] [ ] [ ] [ ]

GLASSES OF WATER
STRESS 1 2 3 4 5 6 7 8 9 10

Notes

November 2016

Monday 7
Breakfast | Lunch | Dinner

WorkOut Time | ● LOWER BODY | ● CORE | ● UPPER BODY | ● CARDIO | ● STRETCH | ● OTHER

GLASSES OF WATER
STRESS 1 2 3 4 5 6 7 8 9 10

Tuesday 8
Breakfast | Lunch | Dinner

WorkOut Time | ● LOWER BODY | ● CORE | ● UPPER BODY | ● CARDIO | ● STRETCH | ● OTHER

GLASSES OF WATER
STRESS 1 2 3 4 5 6 7 8 9 10

Wednesday 9
Breakfast | Lunch | Dinner

WorkOut Time | ● LOWER BODY | ● CORE | ● UPPER BODY | ● CARDIO | ● STRETCH | ● OTHER

GLASSES OF WATER
STRESS 1 2 3 4 5 6 7 8 9 10

Thursday 10
Breakfast | Lunch | Dinner

WorkOut Time | ● LOWER BODY | ● CORE | ● UPPER BODY | ● CARDIO | ● STRETCH | ● OTHER

GLASSES OF WATER
STRESS 1 2 3 4 5 6 7 8 9 10

Friday 11

	Breakfast	Lunch	Dinner

WorkOut ● LOWER BODY ● CORE ● UPPER BODY ● CARDIO ● STRETCH ● OTHER

Time

GLASSES OF WATER

STRESS 1 2 3 4 5 6 7 8 9 10

Saturday 12

	Breakfast	Lunch	Dinner

WorkOut ● LOWER BODY ● CORE ● UPPER BODY ● CARDIO ● STRETCH ● OTHER

Time

GLASSES OF WATER

STRESS 1 2 3 4 5 6 7 8 9 10

Sunday 13

	Breakfast	Lunch	Dinner

WorkOut ● LOWER BODY ● CORE ● UPPER BODY ● CARDIO ● STRETCH ● OTHER

Time

GLASSES OF WATER

STRESS 1 2 3 4 5 6 7 8 9 10

Notes

Monday 14

Breakfast	Lunch	Dinner

WorkOut ● LOWER BODY ● CORE ● UPPER BODY ● CARDIO ● STRETCH ● OTHER

Time [ ] [ ] [ ] [ ] [ ] [ ]

GLASSES OF WATER

STRESS 1 2 3 4 5 6 7 8 9 10

Tuesday 15

Breakfast	Lunch	Dinner

WorkOut ● LOWER BODY ● CORE ● UPPER BODY ● CARDIO ● STRETCH ● OTHER

Time [ ] [ ] [ ] [ ] [ ] [ ]

GLASSES OF WATER

STRESS 1 2 3 4 5 6 7 8 9 10

Wednesday 16

Breakfast	Lunch	Dinner

WorkOut ● LOWER BODY ● CORE ● UPPER BODY ● CARDIO ● STRETCH ● OTHER

Time [ ] [ ] [ ] [ ] [ ] [ ]

GLASSES OF WATER

STRESS 1 2 3 4 5 6 7 8 9 10

Thursday 17

Breakfast	Lunch	Dinner

WorkOut ● LOWER BODY ● CORE ● UPPER BODY ● CARDIO ● STRETCH ● OTHER

Time [ ] [ ] [ ] [ ] [ ] [ ]

GLASSES OF WATER

STRESS 1 2 3 4 5 6 7 8 9 10

November 2016

Friday 18

Breakfast	Lunch	Dinner

WorkOut ●LOWER BODY ●CORE ●UPPER BODY ●CARDIO ●STRETCH ●OTHER
Time

GLASSES OF WATER

STRESS 1 2 3 4 5 6 7 8 9 10

Saturday 19

Breakfast	Lunch	Dinner

WorkOut ●LOWER BODY ●CORE ●UPPER BODY ●CARDIO ●STRETCH ●OTHER
Time

GLASSES OF WATER

STRESS 1 2 3 4 5 6 7 8 9 10

Sunday 20

Breakfast	Lunch	Dinner

WorkOut ●LOWER BODY ●CORE ●UPPER BODY ●CARDIO ●STRETCH ●OTHER
Time

GLASSES OF WATER

STRESS 1 2 3 4 5 6 7 8 9 10

Notes

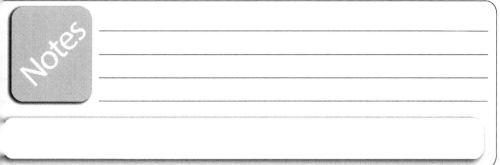

November 2016

Monday 21

	Breakfast	Lunch	Dinner

WorkOut Time ● LOWER BODY ● CORE ● UPPER BODY ● CARDIO ● STRETCH ● OTHER

GLASSES OF WATER

STRESS 1 2 3 4 5 6 7 8 9 10

Tuesday 22

	Breakfast	Lunch	Dinner

WorkOut Time ● LOWER BODY ● CORE ● UPPER BODY ● CARDIO ● STRETCH ● OTHER

GLASSES OF WATER

STRESS 1 2 3 4 5 6 7 8 9 10

Wednesday 23

	Breakfast	Lunch	Dinner

WorkOut Time ● LOWER BODY ● CORE ● UPPER BODY ● CARDIO ● STRETCH ● OTHER

GLASSES OF WATER

STRESS 1 2 3 4 5 6 7 8 9 10

Thursday 24

	Breakfast	Lunch	Dinner

WorkOut Time ● LOWER BODY ● CORE ● UPPER BODY ● CARDIO ● STRETCH ● OTHER

GLASSES OF WATER

STRESS 1 2 3 4 5 6 7 8 9 10

November

Friday 25

Breakfast	Lunch	Dinner

WorkOut ● LOWER BODY ● CORE ● UPPER BODY ● CARDIO ● STRETCH ● OTHER

Time

GLASSES OF WATER

STRESS 1 2 3 4 5 6 7 8 9 10

Saturday 26

Breakfast	Lunch	Dinner

WorkOut ● LOWER BODY ● CORE ● UPPER BODY ● CARDIO ● STRETCH ● OTHER

Time

GLASSES OF WATER

STRESS 1 2 3 4 5 6 7 8 9 10

Sunday 27

Breakfast	Lunch	Dinner

WorkOut ● LOWER BODY ● CORE ● UPPER BODY ● CARDIO ● STRETCH ● OTHER

Time

GLASSES OF WATER

STRESS 1 2 3 4 5 6 7 8 9 10

Notes

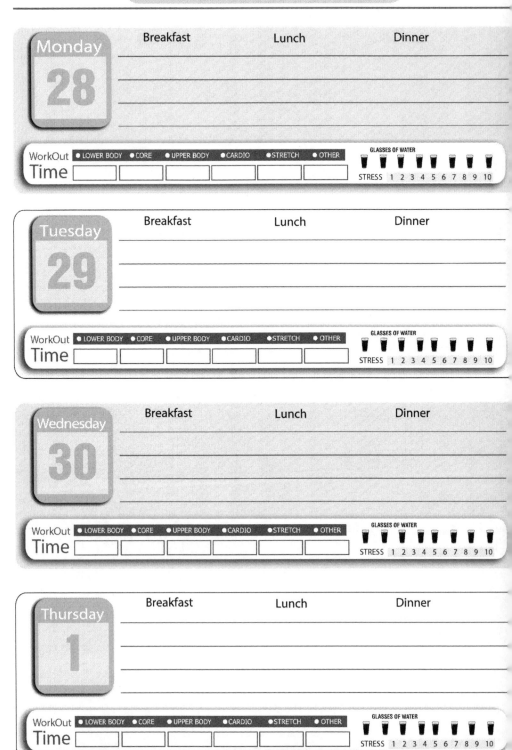

Monday
28

Breakfast Lunch Dinner

WorkOut Time
● LOWER BODY ● CORE ● UPPER BODY ● CARDIO ● STRETCH ● OTHER

GLASSES OF WATER
STRESS 1 2 3 4 5 6 7 8 9 10

Tuesday
29

Breakfast Lunch Dinner

WorkOut Time
● LOWER BODY ● CORE ● UPPER BODY ● CARDIO ● STRETCH ● OTHER

GLASSES OF WATER
STRESS 1 2 3 4 5 6 7 8 9 10

Wednesday
30

Breakfast Lunch Dinner

WorkOut Time
● LOWER BODY ● CORE ● UPPER BODY ● CARDIO ● STRETCH ● OTHER

GLASSES OF WATER
STRESS 1 2 3 4 5 6 7 8 9 10

Thursday
1

Breakfast Lunch Dinner

WorkOut Time
● LOWER BODY ● CORE ● UPPER BODY ● CARDIO ● STRETCH ● OTHER

GLASSES OF WATER
STRESS 1 2 3 4 5 6 7 8 9 10

December 2016

Friday 2

	Breakfast	Lunch	Dinner

WorkOut ● LOWER BODY ● CORE ● UPPER BODY ● CARDIO ● STRETCH ● OTHER

Time

GLASSES OF WATER

STRESS 1 2 3 4 5 6 7 8 9 10

Saturday 3

	Breakfast	Lunch	Dinner

WorkOut ● LOWER BODY ● CORE ● UPPER BODY ● CARDIO ● STRETCH ● OTHER

Time

GLASSES OF WATER

STRESS 1 2 3 4 5 6 7 8 9 10

Sunday 4

	Breakfast	Lunch	Dinner

WorkOut ● LOWER BODY ● CORE ● UPPER BODY ● CARDIO ● STRETCH ● OTHER

Time

GLASSES OF WATER

STRESS 1 2 3 4 5 6 7 8 9 10

This Month's Measurements:

Waist
Neck
Biceps
Chest
Hips
Thighs

Month Progress Report

Current Weight:

Notes:

Monday
5

Breakfast   Lunch   Dinner

WorkOut ● LOWER BODY ● CORE ● UPPER BODY ● CARDIO ● STRETCH ● OTHER

Time

GLASSES OF WATER

STRESS 1 2 3 4 5 6 7 8 9 10

Tuesday
6

Breakfast   Lunch   Dinner

WorkOut ● LOWER BODY ● CORE ● UPPER BODY ● CARDIO ● STRETCH ● OTHER

Time

GLASSES OF WATER

STRESS 1 2 3 4 5 6 7 8 9 10

Wednesday
7

Breakfast   Lunch   Dinner

WorkOut ● LOWER BODY ● CORE ● UPPER BODY ● CARDIO ● STRETCH ● OTHER

Time

GLASSES OF WATER

STRESS 1 2 3 4 5 6 7 8 9 10

Thursday
8

Breakfast   Lunch   Dinner

WorkOut ● LOWER BODY ● CORE ● UPPER BODY ● CARDIO ● STRETCH ● OTHER

Time

GLASSES OF WATER

STRESS 1 2 3 4 5 6 7 8 9 10

Friday 9

Breakfast | Lunch | Dinner

WorkOut Time ● LOWER BODY ● CORE ● UPPER BODY ● CARDIO ● STRETCH ● OTHER

GLASSES OF WATER

STRESS 1 2 3 4 5 6 7 8 9 10

Saturday 10

Breakfast | Lunch | Dinner

WorkOut Time ● LOWER BODY ● CORE ● UPPER BODY ● CARDIO ● STRETCH ● OTHER

GLASSES OF WATER

STRESS 1 2 3 4 5 6 7 8 9 10

Sunday 11

Breakfast | Lunch | Dinner

WorkOut Time ● LOWER BODY ● CORE ● UPPER BODY ● CARDIO ● STRETCH ● OTHER

GLASSES OF WATER

STRESS 1 2 3 4 5 6 7 8 9 10

Notes

December 2016

Monday 12

Breakfast   Lunch   Dinner

WorkOut ● LOWER BODY ● CORE ● UPPER BODY ● CARDIO ● STRETCH ● OTHER
Time

GLASSES OF WATER
STRESS 1 2 3 4 5 6 7 8 9 10

Tuesday 13

Breakfast   Lunch   Dinner

WorkOut ● LOWER BODY ● CORE ● UPPER BODY ● CARDIO ● STRETCH ● OTHER
Time

GLASSES OF WATER
STRESS 1 2 3 4 5 6 7 8 9 10

Wednesday 14

Breakfast   Lunch   Dinner

WorkOut ● LOWER BODY ● CORE ● UPPER BODY ● CARDIO ● STRETCH ● OTHER
Time

GLASSES OF WATER
STRESS 1 2 3 4 5 6 7 8 9 10

Thursday 15

Breakfast   Lunch   Dinner

WorkOut ● LOWER BODY ● CORE ● UPPER BODY ● CARDIO ● STRETCH ● OTHER
Time

GLASSES OF WATER
STRESS 1 2 3 4 5 6 7 8 9 10

Friday 16

Breakfast	Lunch	Dinner

WorkOut ● LOWER BODY ● CORE ● UPPER BODY ● CARDIO ● STRETCH ● OTHER

Time [ ] [ ] [ ] [ ] [ ] [ ]

GLASSES OF WATER

STRESS 1 2 3 4 5 6 7 8 9 10

Saturday 17

Breakfast	Lunch	Dinner

WorkOut ● LOWER BODY ● CORE ● UPPER BODY ● CARDIO ● STRETCH ● OTHER

Time [ ] [ ] [ ] [ ] [ ] [ ]

GLASSES OF WATER

STRESS 1 2 3 4 5 6 7 8 9 10

Sunday 18

Breakfast	Lunch	Dinner

WorkOut ● LOWER BODY ● CORE ● UPPER BODY ● CARDIO ● STRETCH ● OTHER

Time [ ] [ ] [ ] [ ] [ ] [ ]

GLASSES OF WATER

STRESS 1 2 3 4 5 6 7 8 9 10

Notes

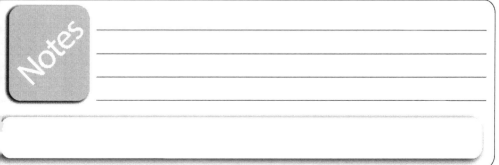

Monday
19

Breakfast   Lunch   Dinner

WorkOut ● LOWER BODY ● CORE ● UPPER BODY ● CARDIO ● STRETCH ● OTHER

Time

GLASSES OF WATER

STRESS 1 2 3 4 5 6 7 8 9 10

Tuesday
20

Breakfast   Lunch   Dinner

WorkOut ● LOWER BODY ● CORE ● UPPER BODY ● CARDIO ● STRETCH ● OTHER

Time

GLASSES OF WATER

STRESS 1 2 3 4 5 6 7 8 9 10

Wednesday
21

Breakfast   Lunch   Dinner

WorkOut ● LOWER BODY ● CORE ● UPPER BODY ● CARDIO ● STRETCH ● OTHER

Time

GLASSES OF WATER

STRESS 1 2 3 4 5 6 7 8 9 10

Thursday
22

Breakfast   Lunch   Dinner

WorkOut ● LOWER BODY ● CORE ● UPPER BODY ● CARDIO ● STRETCH ● OTHER

Time

GLASSES OF WATER

STRESS 1 2 3 4 5 6 7 8 9 10

Friday 23

Breakfast	Lunch	Dinner

WorkOut ●LOWER BODY ●CORE ●UPPER BODY ●CARDIO ●STRETCH ●OTHER

Time

GLASSES OF WATER

STRESS 1 2 3 4 5 6 7 8 9 10

Saturday 24

Breakfast	Lunch	Dinner

WorkOut ●LOWER BODY ●CORE ●UPPER BODY ●CARDIO ●STRETCH ●OTHER

Time

GLASSES OF WATER

STRESS 1 2 3 4 5 6 7 8 9 10

Sunday 25

Breakfast	Lunch	Dinner

WorkOut ●LOWER BODY ●CORE ●UPPER BODY ●CARDIO ●STRETCH ●OTHER

Time

GLASSES OF WATER

STRESS 1 2 3 4 5 6 7 8 9 10

Notes

December 2016

Monday 26
Breakfast | Lunch | Dinner

WorkOut ● LOWER BODY ● CORE ● UPPER BODY ● CARDIO ● STRETCH ● OTHER
Time
GLASSES OF WATER
STRESS 1 2 3 4 5 6 7 8 9 10

Tuesday 27
Breakfast | Lunch | Dinner

WorkOut ● LOWER BODY ● CORE ● UPPER BODY ● CARDIO ● STRETCH ● OTHER
Time
GLASSES OF WATER
STRESS 1 2 3 4 5 6 7 8 9 10

Wednesday 28
Breakfast | Lunch | Dinner

WorkOut ● LOWER BODY ● CORE ● UPPER BODY ● CARDIO ● STRETCH ● OTHER
Time
GLASSES OF WATER
STRESS 1 2 3 4 5 6 7 8 9 10

Thursday 29
Breakfast | Lunch | Dinner

WorkOut ● LOWER BODY ● CORE ● UPPER BODY ● CARDIO ● STRETCH ● OTHER
Time
GLASSES OF WATER
STRESS 1 2 3 4 5 6 7 8 9 10

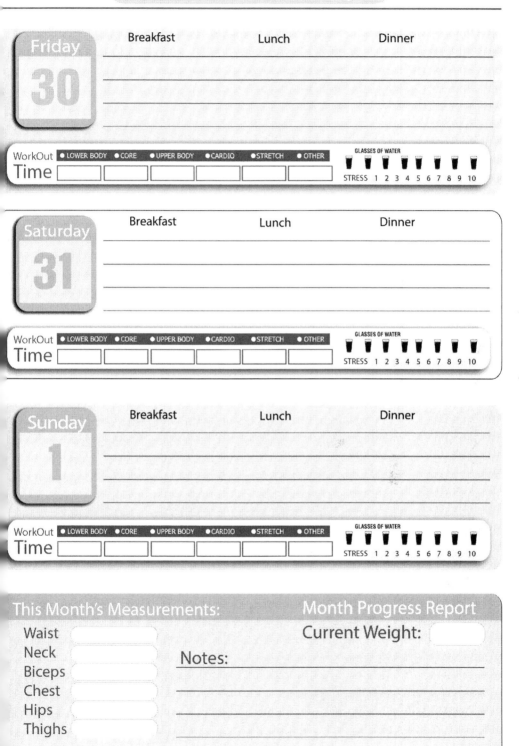

Made in the USA
Middletown, DE
29 December 2016